ALCOHOL AND SEXUALITY

Sexual Medicine, Volume 7

HAROLD I. LIEF, M.D., SERIES EDITOR

VOLUMES IN THE SERIES

Lief and Hoch: **International Research in Sexology, 1984**
Selected Papers from the Fifth World Congress

Segraves and Haeberle: **Emerging Dimensions of Sexology, 1984**
Selected Papers from the Sixth World Congress

Burgess and Hartman: **Sexual Exploitation of Patients by Health Professionals, 1986**

Ross: **Psychovenereology, 1986**

Pope and Bouhoutsos: **Sexual Intimacy between Therapists and Patients, 1986**

Persky: **Psychoendocrinology of Human Sexual Behavior, 1987**

Schuster: **Alcohol and Sexuality, 1988**

ALCOHOL AND SEXUALITY

Carlotta Schuster, M.D.

PRAEGER

New York
Westport, Connecticut
London

Library of Congress Cataloging-in-Publication Data

Schuster, Carlotta.
Alcohol and sexuality.

(Sexual medicine series ; v. 7)
Includes bibliographies and index.
1. Alcohol—Physiological effect. 2. Sexual disorders. 3. Alcoholism—Psychological aspects. 4. Alcoholics—Sexual behavior. I. Title. II. Series: Sexual medicine ; v. 7. [DNLM: 1. Alcohol Drinking. 2. Alcoholism. 3. Sex Behavior—drug effects. 4. Sex Disorders—chemically induced. W1 SE99F v.7 / WM 274 S395a]
QP801.A3S36 1988 616.86'1 87-7182
ISBN 0-275-92559-5 (alk. paper)

Library of Congress Catalog Card Number: 87-7182

ISBN: 0-275-92559-5

First published in 1988

Praeger Publishers, One Madison Avenue, New York, NY 10010
A division of Greenwood Press, Inc.

Printed in the United States of America

The paper used in this book complies with the Permanent Paper Standard issued by the National Information Standards Organization (Z39.48-1984).

10 9 8 7 6 5 4 3 2 1

To David and Amanda

Contents

Foreword

The effect of alcohol on sexual behavior is a central theme of Dr. Carlotta Schuster's monograph. The effects of acute or chronic alcohol ingestion on the sexual responses of heterosexual and gay men and women are reviewed in detail. She brings to life the research reports by presenting a series of illuminating case vignettes.

Dr. Schuster reminds us of Macbeth wherein the porter says, "It (alcohol) provokes and unprovokes: it provokes the desire, but it takes away the performance." It is amazing how many scores of scientific projects have been mounted to test the accuracy of those immortal words. These are described and summarized in this volume, so the reader can ascertain the conditions and circumstances that change, modify or confirm Shakespeare's observation.

On reading Dr. Schuster's monograph, it gradually dawned on me, a student of sexual function and dysfunction, and not, like Dr. Schuster, an expert on alcoholism, that there are striking parallels and ways of looking at these two facets of life, alcohol and sex. Both can be, and generally are, a source of great pleasure, satisfaction, and enhancement of living, or they can be the cause of intense misery, unhappiness, loss of psychological or physiological function, of intense craving, loss of control and of self-respect, and enormous disruption of intimate and loving relationships.

The complexity of both alcohol addiction and sexual behavior are almost mind-boggling. Think of the interplay among these diverse elements. One must consider on the *biological* side: genetic factors interacting with constitutional influences, such as fetal hormones and enzymes, brain anatomy and physiology, including the role of the endorphins, of the brain messengers (neurotransmitters), hormones, especially those of the hypothalamic-pituitary-gonadal axis, the various bodily systems, for example the neurological and circulatory involved in both alcohol and sex, the gastrointestinal system, including the liver, in alcoholism, and the genito-urinary system in sex; *psychological* factors: personality conflicts or traits (a controversial subject), motivational states, for example alcohol and sex-seeking desires, influence of cognition, for example internal scripting, including attitudes, expectations and emotions; *interpersonal* aspects; influence and reactions to spouse, parents, and other family members, peer pressure; *cultural* factors, such as shame-inducing social attitudes, cultural norms, legal restrictions and penalties. Finally, the *behavioral expression* of these complex interactive factors and behavior. As suggested above, the range of behavior is enormous, from total abstinence from either alcohol or sex, or both, to their use to enhance the pleasures of living, and, at the other end of the spectrum, alcohol and sexual behaviors may become self-destructive. Addiction is not restricted to alcoholism; sexual addiction occurs in a variety of ways as well.

The study of alcohol use or of sexual behavior involves investigation of the factors mentioned above. But, in addition, one can benefit from looking at these two pleasure-pain pursuits demographically (race, ethnic group, age, sex, etc.) and developmentally. Sexual behavior changes, sometimes dramatically, throughout the life cycle from conception to death, and alcohol use has its developmental and historical side as well, for example, the differences between types of alcoholism manifested by early onset (before age 25) and later onset (Cloninger, 1987).

An extensive, let alone an exhaustive, analysis of the complexities of alcohol use and sexuality and their comparison merits a much longer essay, but since this approach supplements that followed by Dr. Schuster, allow me to set forth in an abbreviated fashion a few illustrations enlarging on the topics addressed above.

INHERITANCE

We know more about this in alcoholism than in sex. "Children who are reared by alcoholic adoptive parents are no more likely to become alcoholic themselves than other children; however, children of alcoholic biologic parents are more likely than other children to misuse alcohol, even when they are separated from their biological parents in infancy and placed in stable adoptive homes'' (Cloninger, 1987). It appears as if the incidence of alcoholism is four to five times higher in the sons of alcoholics than in the sons of non-alcoholic fathers regardless of their rearing. While we know some things about the inheritance of intersexuality (ambiguous sex organs and genitalia), we know practically nothing about the inheritance of sexual disorders, either paraphilias or of sexual dysfunctions, assuming that there may be still unknown genetic factors in the inheritance of sexual behavior (an assumption that may not necessarily turn out to be true). This came home to me when I thought about a woman with a total absence of sexual desire whom I was interviewing for a research project. She reported that she had three other sisters, among a total of seven sisters, who had the same problem, and so did her mother. Inheritance or environmental? Nature or nurture? There were no immediately apparent environmental factors, and indeed this woman previously had had a period of good sexual functioning for eight years.

CONSTITUTIONAL FACTORS

What happens between conception and birth is termed ''constitutional.'' In contrast to our ignorance about heredity, we know more about sexual develolpment as a consequence of constitutional factors than we do about these possible etiologic factors in alcohol use and abuse. To be sure, there is growing evidence of the ill effects of the mother's drinking on the offspring in the so-called ''fetal alcohol syndrome,'' but the connection with later alcohol abuse is obscure. On the other hand, to take two examples, there is a wealth of evidence about the significance of fetal testicular secretions of androgen on the XY fetus between roughly the twelfth and twentieth fetal week. In its absence, or in the failure of the ''key lock'' mechanism where receptor cells are unavailable or working improperly, we see the ''androgen insensitivity syndrome'' with its feminizing effects. The opposite occurs as well. In an XX fetus, an excess of androgen secreted by the fetal adrenals has masculizing effects. This oversimplified account is made to suggest the importance of fetal factors in the later development of sexuality. Similar speculations about fetal potentials for the development of homosexuality, and perhaps even of transsexualism, are now current.

NEUROTRANSMITTERS

In an intriguing article, Cloninger posits three genetically independent dimensions of personality that are mediated by the three main neuromodulator systems in the brain. He links "novelty-seeking" ("frequent exploratory activity and intense exhilaration in response to novel or appetitive stimuli") with the dopamine system "leading to behavioral activation. Alcohol-seeking behavior is considered to be a special instance of exploratory appetitive behavior."

A second personality dimension is "harm avoidance" (an intense response to aversive stimuli leading to an inhibition of behavior in order to avoid punishment, frustration or harm). This system seems to reduce anxiety and is dependent on the second major neuromodulator system, namely serotonin. The person who has high harm avoidance seeks out additional ways to reduce anxiety, including alcohol, and, in Cloninger's view, is susceptible to loss of control.

A third dimension, "reward dependence," is linked to the maintenance of behavior and is mediated by the third neuromodulator system, namely norepinephrine. This is implicated in the tolerance of alcohol.

No one has suggested a similar schema for sexuality, but we do know that sexual desire particularly seems mediated by the dopamine system. It is not too far-fetched to think of "novelty-seeking" and "intense exhilaration" in response to appetitive stimuli in the context of sexual approach behavior. Indeed, Frank Beach (1976) and John Money (1980) have called this "proception" ("the phase of invitation, of solicitation and seduction, and of attraction"). We know that dopamine agonists, such as certain antidepressants, alcohol itself, amphetamines, cocaine, and opiates, facilitate both alcohol and sexual-seeking behaviors.

On the other hand, serotonin activity inhibits such behavior. It is known that serotonin diminishes sexual interest and activity. Alcohol, a dopamine agonist, is a serotonin antagonist (blocks serotonin activity) and thus "inhibits the inhibition," the net effect being a decrease in the ability to predict punishment or the frustration of rewards, and a decrease in self-protective behavior. Again the parallel between alcohol and sexual-seeking and maintaining behaviors are suggestive.

Since the third neuromodulator, the norepinephrine system, is linked closely with activities of the locus coeruleus in the pons, and we know the importance of that structure in anxiety, panic reactions and phobias, one can speculate that overactivity of this system is involved with sexual phobias and aversion, and underactivity with sexual and alcohol addictions.

HORMONES

The effects of alcohol on the hypothalamic-pituitary-gonadal axis is described by Dr. Schuster, so I will not elaborate here. The decrease in testosterone is mediated by more than one mechanism, for example a direct effect on the brain and a direct effect on liver cells and enzymes. This is of particular importance since sexual desire is androgen driven in women as well as in men (Persky, 1987).

OTHER BODY SYSTEMS

Alcohol abuse can have a direct effect on the brain, the liver, and on the upper end of the gastrointestinal tract, the nerves themselves, and, less significantly, on other parts of the body. Sexual activity may be affected by the alcohol-mediated cerebral defects of cognition, judgment, memory and decreased inhibition, by neuropathy affecting penile enervation and hence sensation, and by any serious illness, especially those associated with alcoholism, such as diabetes and hypertension, causing physical dysfunction, or at least pain and fatigue. These are some of the ways that alcohol abuse and sexual behavior interdigitate.

INTRAPSYCHIC FACTORS

A controversy surrounds the idea that personality problems are causative factors in alcoholism. Overdeveloped consciences, repressed homosexual impulses, and excessive dependency are just three of the theories that have had advocates for many years. Recent research has failed to find predictive power among personality problems. Cloninger, as indicated above, has postulated more sophisticated motivation and learning dimensions, "novelty-seeking," "harm avoidance," and "reward dependence" in his attempt to develop a neurobiological learning model. These are exciting ideas, and, if it does nothing else, it conveys suggestions for additional research. The relation between personality factors and sexual behavior is mostly unexplored, although an approach is to be found in the ideas of Avodah Offit (in press). She singles out five major personality dimensions that have maladaptive sexual consequences:

1. Restricted ability to express genuine warm and tender emotions.
2. Difficulty with rejection or criticism.
3. Difficulties with exhibiting, either too little or too much. Entities that may or may not be exhibited include reason, order, emotions, possessions, body, protectiveness, and the need to be protected.
4. Difficulties with perception of authority.
5. Difficulty with basic self-esteem.

She feels that these are the main areas to be dealt with in the personal and interpersonal therapy of the sexual dysfunctions. It would be interesting to take these five major personality dimensions and apply them to alcohol abuse. Of course, the immediate methodological problem is the terrible distortion created by retrospective analysis. What alcoholic does not suffer from deficient self-esteem?

OTHER INTRAPSYCHIC DIMENSIONS

Because Dr. Schuster describes the research studies dealing with the effects of expectancy as part of cognitive scripting for anticipated behavior and also of emotions on the interplay between alcohol and sex, I will illustrate the significance of intrapsychic factors by briefly discussing stress, anxiety, and alcohol. If a person has imbibed a certain amount (and the amount is, of course, important) of alcohol, and is in a sexual situation, and is also undergoing a certain amount of stress causing varying amounts of anxiety (note that the quantification of alcohol, stress, and anxiety is necessary), how do these play into one another? One can see that this is a complex situation. For one thing, what is stress to one person may be neutral or even exciting (facilitating, stimulating, enhancing) to another. Second, low amounts of stress usually enhance sexual arousal, and high degrees of stress decrease it (less arousal than a response to a neutral stimulus). Third, alcohol, or even its expectation, in low doses enhances sexual arousal, and in high doses decreases it. The complexity of the interaction among these variables makes it clear that sexual desire and arousal is greatly influenced by the setting and circumstances in which drinking occurs.

INTERPERSONAL FACTORS

One has only to point to Al-Anon, Alateen, or the self-help group Adult Children of Alcoholics to underscore the importance of family members to the alcoholic. Since most adult sexual activity involves a partner, I do not have to belabor the significance of relationships and the common thread between the two behaviors. One illustrative study found that 80 percent of the alcoholics reported that their partners were not interested in sex when they were drunk.

Peer pressure to drink and to engage in sex. Are there not striking parallels? Pressure to belong, to be accepted to the group, to prove one's masculinity or femininity, to show that one is grown up and is no longer a kid, not to be regarded as a "nerd," etc. Is it any wonder that alcohol and sex are a twosome, sometimes a "gruesome twosome" among teenagers.

SOCIAL AND CULTURAL FACTORS

Cultural norms certainly influence engaging in sex outside of marriage, as well as the frequency and intensity of drinking. Compare a society that promotes wine drinking among its teenagers and a somewhat liberal attitude toward premarital sex with, let us say, by way of example, a Southern Baptist upbringing where it is often regarded as sinful to drink, smoke, dance, have sex before marriage, or even play cards. Of course, rebellion against these standards is not unknown, but they still have an influence, for the rebel often goes overboard in the opposite direction, as in the case of the minister's daughter taking up prostitution.

Social circumstances play an important role in both drinking and sex. Its availability, its facilitation by advertising and by institutions that cater to the need for both, such as bars, massage parlors and dance halls, increase their consumption, whereas inhibition is created by religious or health-promoting groups. It is interesting to note, for example, the marked decrease in unsafe sex among groups of homosexuals after sufficient education about the perils of AIDS.

Social norms have an important influence on both drinking and sex, but even these have their limits. Prohibition did not end the use of alcohol or have a material effect on the amount of alcoholism. Rigid church doctrine did not prevent one of three young women in puritan New England from becoming pregnant before marriage, nor have church, social and legal sanctions against homosexuality made it disappear.

BEHAVIOR

An analysis of sex and alcohol-related behavior makes up the bulk of Dr. Schuster's monograph. I will restrict myself to a few general comments. I look for parallels in alcohol and sex-seeking behavior, in the search for novelty and excitement, in what creates "set maintenance" and "set breaking" behaviors, that is, what influences the need to maintain a set of behaviors, whether this be drinking or sex, versus the need to break out of the mold and upset the equilibrium? Finally, are there parallels in the addictive aspects of drinking and sex, the compulsive behaviors and fantasies that precede and accompany such behaviors? Are there not similar mechanisms of defense, for example denial, rationalization, social withdrawal, etc.? Do they reduce anxiety in similar or different ways?

DEMOGRAPHIC FACTORS

The comparison of sexual behavior and alcohol-consuming behavior in different racial, ethnic, socioeconomic and age groups would make a fascinating study remaining, so far as I know, to be undertaken. Research, on socioeconomic status, has been reported with both sets of behaviors, so that it would require a review of the literature to pull together salient comparisons and new research to fill in the gaps. However, it would be more valuable to study *the same groups at the same time*, and to make it contemporaneous rather than retrospective, for only in this way can we be sure of the validity of comparative data.

LIFE CYCLE EVENTS

Sex has been studied throughout the life cycle (see, for example, Gadpaille's *The Cycles of Sex*), and there are studies of early and late onset of alcoholism, and studies of drinking among adolescents, but I do not believe that anyone in reviewing the literature has integrated them, let alone set up specific research projects.

In reading Dr. Schuster's valuable review of the literature dealing with sex and alcohol, one cannot help but be impressed with the complexities of the subject and the challenges to make sense of it. She helps us by separating acute from chronic alcohol consumption, social drinking from alcoholism, the effects of varying dosage levels in different groups, the importance of expectancies (cognitive scripting), the contributions of pharmacologic and psychological processes, and applying these to a comparison of men and women, of heterosexuals and homosexuals. Through her case histories, she illustrates the various methods of treatment and case management. As the editor of the series on Sexual Medicine, I welcome this addition to the series. I believe that the volume will be of great interest to all students of human behavior, as well as counselors and therapists of alcohol related and of sexual problems, and will encourage researchers to develop protocols for the prospective studies still needed.

Harold I. Lief, M.D.

REFERENCES

Beach, F.A. 1976. "Sexual Attractivity, Proceptivity and Receptivity in Female Mammals," Hormones and Behaviors, Vol. 7, pp. 105-138.

Cloninger, C.R. 1987. "Neurogenetic Adaptive Mechanisms in Alcoholism," Science, Vol. 236, p. 410.

Gadpaille, Warren J. 1975. *The Cycles of Sex* (L. Freeman, ed.), New York: Charles Scribner's Sons.

Money, J. 1980. *Love and Lovesickness: Science of Sex, Gender Difference and Pair-Bonding*. Baltimore: The Johns Hopkins University Press.

Offit, A. (in press). "Psychiatric Disorders and Sexual Dysfunctions." In *Treatment of Psychosexual Disorders* (H. Lief, ed.), Washington, D.C.: American Psychiatric Association.

Persky, H. 1987. *Psychoendocrinology of Human Sexual Behavior*. Vol. 6 in series on Sexual Medicine. New York: Praeger.

Introduction

When it was suggested that I write this monograph, I felt considerable apprehension about the availability of literature that bridged the fields of substance abuse and sexuality. Although researchers and clinicians involved in the study and treatment of human sexuality considered the drug histories of their patients, it is only recently that substance abuse specialists have devoted much thought to the sexual effects of alcohol and other drugs.

A great deal of earlier material about sexuality and alcohol is anecdotal. Conclusions are based on psychodynamic formulations which, in most instances, have been contradicted by more recent data.

In this book, social and pathological drinking in males is dealt with in separate chapters in order to emphasize the differences between the physiological effects of single drinking events and alcoholism. Because men and women have different sets of hormonal and emotional reactions to sex and alcohol, this book is further divided into chapters dealing with sexual response in female social drinkers and sexual response in alcoholic women.

Most rehabilitation centers now treat larger numbers of polysubstance abusers. Formerly, alcoholics were separated from "drug addicts." Each group was treated in centers with distinct and conflicting program philosophies. In the past ten years, with an explosion of knowledge about the neurochemistry of addiction along with the availability of self-help groups such as Narcotics Anonymous and Cocaine Anonymous in addition to Alcoholics Anonymous, there has been a blending of treatment approaches and a merging of populations in treatment centers.

Furthermore, about half the alcoholic patients under 40 are cross-addicted. This has afforded me the opportunity to make clinical observations about the ways in which drugs other than alcohol influence human sexual response. Chapter 5 comprises a review of the literature about the sexual effects of barbiturates and benzodiazepines (which are similar to alcohol, as might be expected) as well as cocaine and amphetamines, opioids, and marijuana.

All of the chapters about alcoholism or other substance abuse contain case histories. These are based on clinical experience derived from my work in the substance abuse service at Silver Hill Foundation, which is a private, nonprofit, general psychiatric hospital. Each of the cases is a composite of the stories of several patients with similar clinical features. In addition, names, locations, occupations, and ages have been changed to prevent identification.

I would like to thank the staff and patients of Silver Hill Foundation for providing me with whatever substance abuse expertise I possess. Mildred Eisele warrants special acknowledgment for her invaluable assistance in locating journal articles. I would also like to thank Harold Lief, M.D., for having introduced me, 20 years ago, to research efforts in the field of human sexuality.

1

The Effect of Alcohol on Sexual Response of Male Social Drinkers

INTRODUCTION

According to a recent Gallup survey, 39 percent of the male teenage population, 75 percent of male college students, and 72 percent of adult men drink alcoholic beverages (Gallup 1986). There is surprisingly little information available about the ways in which this popular drug affects the sexuality of nonalcoholic males.

Prior to the availability of instruments capable of measuring penile tumescence and ejaculatory response, investigators were limited to the reports of their subjects. If researchers and clinicians ventured at all to write about the way in which alcohol influenced the sexual behavior of normal social drinkers, their work was based on case histories and verbal psychological testing. Some correlations were made which are still considered valid, and others have been disproven by experiments using physiological measurements.

It is only recently that hormonal influences of alcohol have been differentiated so that effects of long-term drinking and chronic alcoholism can be separated from those of short-term drinking on a single occasion.

The role of expectancy in sexual behavior while drinking has been taken into account by several investigators. One can summarize the experimental work on expectancy, drinking, and sexual behavior by stating that, at low baseline levels of alcohol consumption, expectancy has a great deal to do with behavior, but, as the amount of alcohol consumed increases, the direct physiological effects of alcohol have a greater influence on erection and ejaculatory capacity.

Throughout the rest of this chapter I will describe earlier and more recent investigations in greater detail. I will refer also to some popular literature because it reflects our society's beliefs and expectations about drinking and sex.

CLINICAL OBSERVATIONS AND CORRELATIONAL INVESTIGATIONS

Physiological

Erection and Ejaculation

While Duncan was being treated most inhospitably, Macbeth's porter made the following remarks regarding the influence of alcohol on sex to another houseguest:

> MACDUFF What three things does drink especially provoke?
>
> PORTER Marry, sir, nose-painting, sleep, and urine. Lechery, sir, it provokes and unprovokes. It provokes the desire, but it takes away the performance. Therefore much drink can be said to be an equivocator with lechery. It makes him and it mars him, it sets him on and it takes him off, it persuades him and disheartens him, makes him stand to and not stand to; in conclusion, equivocates him in a sleep, and, giving him the lie, leaves him.
>
> (*Macbeth*, II, iii, 29-40)

Since Shakespeare's plays often represented beliefs commonly held by his audience, we can surmise that Elizabethans thought alcohol increased desire and interfered frequently with erection.

This opinion has prevailed throughout the centuries. Although alcohol in low doses has been thought to have a disinhibiting effect, leading to promiscuity or, at least, diminished shyness in making sexual overtures, decrease in frequency of intercourse has been ascribed to heavy drinking. In a report about executive life styles, Johnson cited increased fatigue rather than diminution of erection as the cause for decreased intercourse in executives who drank from two to six scotches per day (Johnson 1974). He did suggest that alcohol played a direct role in increasing the frequency of extramarital sex because of enhanced desire but did not speculate about whether this was due to disinhibition, to social expectations about alcohol, or to increased penile tumescence as the result of alcohol. Factors inhibiting extramarital sex, such as romanticism, strong moral values regarding fidelity, and quality of the marital relationship were mentioned but not analyzed.

Masters and Johnson have cited alcohol as "the second most frequent factor in the onset of secondary impotence," which could result from a specific incident involving alcohol ingestion or might accompany a pattern of "excessive alcohol intake" (Masters and Johnson 1970). The onset of secondary impotence occurred after an episode or several episodes of acute alcoholic intake in 35 of a sample of 213 men referred for this complaint to their clinic (Masters and Johnson 1970). These authors also observed that secondary impotence in males in their late forties to fifties "has a higher incidence of direct association with excessive alcohol consumption than with any other single factor." They point out that the trauma of being unable to have or maintain an erection can lead to further tension about sexual performance because their patients had not recognized that alcohol had been the cause of the erectile failure (Masters and Johnson 1966).

Kaplan (1974) states that alcohol increases libido in small doses because of its disinhibiting and anxiety-reducing effect on higher cortical centers. However, in high doses she has found it to produce impotence. Once more, the term "heavy drinking" is not defined, although Kaplan (1974: 89) mentions a typical executive male who drinks "three martinis at lunch, a scotch before he gets on the train and three more drinks at dinner." Impotence seems to refer here to erectile failure. In volume 2 of *The New Sex Therapy*, she speaks explicitly about orgasmic delay in "high doses" (Kaplan 1979). The exact dosage of alcohol is not specified. One assumes that the term "orgasmic delay" refers to ejaculatory dysfunction. The sample size of the population of men observed is not given in either book.

Clinical Observations Regarding the Hormonal Influence of Alcohol on Male Sexuality in Normal Drinkers

Testosterone. Gordon et al. (1976) administered alcohol to nine healthy male volunteers aged 21 to 40 and to two men with a history of alcoholism all of whom had, however, normal liver biopsies. They were hospitalized at the Clinical Research Center of Mount Sinai Hospital for four weeks and given a 15 percent solution of alcohol every three hours around the clock for the entire time. A second group of six normal nonalcoholic subjects was also studied without the aid of liver biopsies but with the same schedule of alcohol dosage. Social drinking was defined as a weekly consumption of alcohol not exceeding 70 g. In the first group a second liver biopsy was performed after four weeks. Metabolic clearance rates of testosterone were determined after 24 to 26 days of alcohol ingestion. It should be noted that the two men in the first group who had a history of alcoholism had abstained from alcohol for two weeks prior to the supervised administration of alcohol.

Results were as follows. In normal men, testosterone is known to be secreted throughout the day in episodic bursts (Weitzman et al. 1975). Exposure to oral doses of alcohol led to an initial dampening of these episodic bursts of testosterone secretion followed by a fall in the plasma level. More prolonged administration (12-24 days) further reduced the mean plasma level of this steroid. All volunteers had adequate nutrition and none lost weight, which excludes nutritional disturbance as a significant factor in the decreased testosterone. The plasma clearance rate of the hormone decreased, which was felt by the authors to be due, at least in part, to decreased protein binding as a result of alcohol. Although it had been demonstrated that chronic alcohol consumption increases the activity of hepatic testosterone A reductase (Rubin et al. 1976), this was not considered to be a contributing factor, because the alcohol was discontinued 12 hours before the clearance measurement and by that time the effect of alcohol on hepatic metabolism would no longer prevail. The authors state further that the findings in these subjects contrast with the findings for liver disease in that patients with cirrhosis have elevated levels of plasma testosterone binding, and decreased metabolic clearance rates of testosterone, that is, the effect of alcohol upon testosterone in cirrhotic males is opposite to its effect on the healthy volunteers in this experiment (Gordon et al. 1976).

It has been established that alcohol decreases serum levels of testosterone after acute as well as chronic exposure (Cicero 1980, 1982; Cicero, Bernstein, and Badger 1978; Ylikahri et al. 1974).

Ylikhari et al. administered 1.5 g/kg alcohol in a 20 percent solution at a constant rate for 3 hours (6 to 9 P.M.) to 10 healthy male students aged 19 to 25. A hangover was experienced the next morning by all subjects. Blood samples for testosterone and for luteinizing hormone were taken when drinking began and 4, 8, 12, 15, and 20 hours later. After 12 to 20 hours, testosterone was decreased and the decrease seemed to correlate with the intensity of the hangover. Plasma LH increased slightly.

Luteinizing hormone. Let's review the normal sequence of events that occurs within the hypophothalamic-pituitary-gonadal axis. The hypothalamus secretes luteinizing hormone releasing hormone (LHRH), which in turn stimulates the pituitary to secrete LH. LH stimulates the production of testosterone by the testes in the male and triggers ovulation in females. A decrease in secretion of testosterone through servoregulation leads to an increased secretion of LHRH and LH. High plasma levels of testosterone would result in negative feedback to the hypothalamus and pituitary, bringing about decreased secretion of LH and LHRH.

Gordon et al. (1976) found that the effect of alcohol on LH secretion in normal men was inconsistent. This supported the hypothesis that alcohol acts directly on the gonads (testosterone was decreased), but it also suggests that alcohol has some hypothalamic-pituitary effects as well in that in some subjects it lowered the LH.

In contrast, Van Thiel has reported elevated LH in some but not all chronic alcoholics presumably due to decreased testosterone (Van Thiel et al. 1974).

Cicero, in a more recent literature review, states that alcohol does not impair the ability of the pituitary to respond to hypothalamic secretion of LHRH in normal nonalcoholic volunteers (Cicero 1982). These statements about pituitary response during acute intoxication in nonalcoholic men suggest that the decrease in testosterone secretion brought about by alcohol is due to a direct effect on the gonads rather than via the hypothalamic-pituitary-gonadal axis. At blood alcohol levels of 50 mg percent or more (the equivalent of three drinks) penile tumescence occurs less readily than it does with lower amounts of alcohol. With blood alcohol levels of 100 mg percent or more, erection is inhibited and "ejaculatory competence is eliminated in many men" (Abel 1985).

Alleged Psychological Influences of Intoxication

Most investigations of the characteristics of drinkers versus nondrinkers have used college student populations. It was usually assumed that both groups were nonalcoholic. Studies of this type usually have not differentiated between men and women (Ratliff and Burkhart 1984) or between normal and abnormal drinking. For example, Rockwell et al. (1973) conclude that college students of both sexes had similar expectations of alcohol as an aphrodisiac (39 percent of 284), but the majority had higher expectations from marijuana. Intercourse was the sexual experience alluded to by 75 percent of the sample. Data on the amount of alcohol or dosage of other drugs is not stated.

Athanasiou, Shaver, and Tavris (1970) received responses from more than 20,000 readers of *Psychology Today.* Forty-five percent of males and 68 percent of women stated that alcohol enhanced enjoyment. Thirteen percent of males and 11 percent of women stated that alcohol had no effect on sexual enjoyment, and 42 percent of males and 21 percent of females reported decreased enjoyment of sex with alcohol. Sex meant intercourse specifically. The amount of alcohol involved was not specified.

Ratliff and Burkhart (1984) chose 70 men and 70 women from a pool of 663 undergraduates at Auburn University who agreed to fill out a brief measure of alcohol intake. Students who did not drink were not included. (Not drinking was defined as less than 6 oz. of absolute alcohol per year.) The study supported previous reports that the need for disinhibition, sensation seeking, and arousal were characteristic of heavy drinkers of both sexes as measured by a Reason for Drinking Scale.

This suggests an expectation on the part of researchers and their subjects that alcohol brings about a degree of social disinhibition sufficient for participation in sexual activities which the absence of alcohol would preclude. In 1967 Beigel stated, without much supporting documentation, that men become more aggressive and "callous about self-control" (p. 510) when they are only "slightly intoxicated." In his often quoted paper, Knight (1937) asserts that drinking results in dissolution of the superego. As Wilson (1977) points out, whether one states it in neurological terms of cortical disinhibition or in psychoanalytic terms, the concept that alcohol results in reduction of judgment leading to disinhibition of sexual behavior has gone largely unchallenged.

Enhanced desire has been attributed to the effects of alcohol (Johnson 1974; Athanasiou, Shaver, and Tavris 1970). It is not clear whether this alleged increase in desire is thought to be due to disinhibition. Goodwin makes the distinction that alcohol "releases" desire as opposed to increasing it (Goodwin 1976).

Violent sexual acts such as rape have been thought to be associated closely with alcohol. Gebhard et al. (1965) interviewed 1,356 sex offenders convicted between 1940 and 1960. Alcohol is thought to be a causative factor through personality deterioration as a result of alcoholism and because of regressive behavior and disinhibition while acutely intoxicated. They documented that, in their sample, alcohol played the largest role in cases of heterosexual aggression against children; here, two-thirds of the men were said to be drunk at the time of the act. Incest, exhibitionism, and homosexual pedophilic acts were associated with intoxication in 20 to 30 percent. Their conclusion was that alcohol intoxication played an especially large role in "the more aberrant crimes such as those that involve children or the use of force" (Gebhard et al. 1965: 762).

Rada (1975) collectd detailed autobiographies from 77 men convicted of rape which revealed that 50 percent of them were drinking at the time of the rape. He states elsewhere, "For the nonalcoholic rapist, drinking prior to the rape allows him to overcome his timidity and fear about social encounters with members of the opposite sex. In this sense, alcohol acts as a psychic muscle-builder."

In a study of 223 male felons about to be released from prison, the role that alcohol had played in their behavior was considered but sexual crimes were not mentioned (Goodwin, Crane, and Guze 1971). Amir (1967) collected data from the files of the Philadelphia Police Department yielding a total of 646 victims of sexual offenses and 1,292 offenders. The discrepency between the numbers of offenders and victims was that, in some cases, more than one offender was involved. In 3 percent of the 646 forcible rape cases, alcohol was present in the offender only. Alcohol was present in both the offender and the victim in 10 percent of the crimes. Alcohol played no role in the majority of the crimes (66 percent or 429 cases). Women who were drunk or drinking in public places were more vulnerable to rape, and the lone black woman was more often victimized than white women. Amir stresses that in the vast majority of cases studied, alcohol was not a factor. He states that "if drinking is assumed to be an accepted kind of leisure among young males, especially in the lower classes, the fact that rape is so infrequently recorded indicates that most men who drink do not commit this offense."

Wilson suggests that offenders stressed their consumption of alcohol to reduce the sentence, which may distort interpretations of data about sex crimes in which the amount of alcohol consumed is known only through the offenders' self-reports (Wilson 1977: 243). In a sense, the presence of alcohol could be said to provide permission for deviance (Lang et al. 1975).

EXPERIMENTAL INVESTIGATION

Effect of Blood Alcohol Level on Penile Tumescence

In 1976 Farkas and Rosen reported the results of an experiment with 16 male college student volunteers who described themselves as moderate drinkers, imbibing alcohol two to three times weekly in unspecified amounts. Sexual arousal elicited by an erotic film was directly determined by two autonomic variables, penile tumescence by means of a mercury-in-rubber strain gauge, and tonic heart rate measured on a Beckman-type RM polygraph. After refraining from alcohol for 24 hours and from food for 3 hours, subjects were brought to one of four blood alcohol levels: 0, 0.025, 0.050, and 0.075 percent. The order in which the alcohol dosage was given was unknown to the subjects, who each attended four sessions. Blood Alcohol Concentration (BAC) was determined by means of a Breathalyzer. Stable heart rate and penile strain gauge recordings were obtained during 10 minutes of incidental music. Following this, the same 15-minute erotic film was used for all four sessions. Penile diameter and tumescence rate were measured. The rate of penile tumescence tended to decrease as BACs increased. There was a curvilinear effect on penile diameter. There was a slight increase in diameter at 0.025 percent, although this trend reversed at higher BACs. At low BACs (less than 0.050 percent) a slight decrease in tumescence rate was associated with the maximum penile diameter increase. However, Farkas and Rosen considered this "a small initial effect when compared with the very considerable inhibition of response present during the very highest levels of the alcohol dose-response curve" (Farkas and Rosen 1976: 270). When BACs were above 0.050 percent, both tumescence rate and diameter diminished rapidly, while tonic heart rate continued to rise. The authors did not comment on the effect that repetition of the same erotic film might have had on their findings.

Effect of Expectancy on Penile Tumescence

Farkas and Rosen (1976) and Masters and Johnson (1970: 163-69) point out that when alcohol prevents formation or maintenance of an erection, this can lead to permanent expectation of erectile failure when vaginal penetration is attempted. In contrast, expectation of enhanced sexual performance in the presence of alcohol may be a prophecy equally self-fulfilling. Rubin and Henson (1976) administered alcohol in varying dosages in order to bring about four different blood alcohol levels in 16 adult male volunteers aged 21 to 29. They were given a placebo, a low dose (0.5-0.6 ml/kg), a moderate dose (1.0-1.2 ml/kg), and a high dose (1.8 ml/kg). Each volunteer viewed four different films twice on two occasions over the course of three sessions. Alcohol was administered only during the second session, with sessions 1 and 3 serving as placebo baselines. Subjects were asked either to relax or to inhibit themselves sexually while watching the films. They were also asked to arouse themselves in the absence of an erotic film. Only the highest dose, producing Blood Alcohol Levels (BALs) between 106 and 156 mg/kg, significantly decreased tumescence measured by penile plethysmography. But even at this dose partial erections exceeding 20 percent of the maximum erection occurred and full erection could be accomplished by a few. Alcohol did not influence subjects' ability to inhibit erection. Rubin and Henson report that 6 of 11 subjects who had believed that alcohol enhanced their sexual functioning prior to the experiment continued to believe it after the experiment was completed.

Wilson (1981) conducted two experiments on expectation of sexual performance with varying doses of alcohol. One study consisted of a sample of nonalcoholics. (The other study, of alcoholic subjects, will be discussed later in this book.) Using 48 undergraduate males as volunteers, Briddell and Wilson (1976) assigned them to eight experimental groups. Each group received one of four dose levels of alcohol and two sets of instruction regarding expectation of alcohol's effect on their sexual performance. They were told either to expect enhanced sexual performance with alcohol or to expect a decrease in sexual functioning. The doses of alcohol were 0.08, 0.05, 0.08, and 1.2 g/kg. This resulted in blood levels of alcohol prior to viewing an erotic film of 0.35, 50, 67, and 95 mg/100 ml. Penile tumescence and electromyelography (EMG) recordings from the subjects' frontalis muscle were monitored continuously throughout the 10-minute erotic film. Sexual imagery evoked by a Thematic Apperception Test (TAT) card administered immediately after the film and self-report of sexual arousal were also measured. The same linear relationship between alcohol dose and penile tumescence existed as in the Farkas and Rosen report, except that there was no increase in the amplitude of tumescence at the low dose. Wilson speculates that this may have been because the BAL produced by this dose was higher in the Briddell and Wilson study than in the study conducted by Farkas and Rosen. The effect of the instructions concerning expectation had no significant effect on penile tumescence. Briddell and Wilson hypothesize that the instructions may have conflicted with the subjects' expectations prior to the experiment. An assessment of prior assumptions "may have served to clarify this issue" (Briddell and Wilson 1976: 232). Muscle tension levels were not altered by alcohol level, failing to support the notion that alcohol reduces muscular tension. No correlations were found between EMG recordings of tension and penile tumescence. The authors suggest that reduction in muscular tension may occur in the later stages of arousal rather than in the initial excitatory phase. In addition, it is speculated that tension reduction may occur in specific muscle regions rather than as a generalized change monitored by the frontalis muscle. The authors note further that sexual imagery as manifested on the TAT was not affected by BAL. There was a significant negative correlation between penile tumescence and the TAT measure. It is suggested by the authors that "subjects who experienced minimal penile tumescence may have attempted to compensate for this perceived 'failure' by loading their TAT stories with erotic content" (p. 233). Subjects correctly identified their states of arousal. Subjective reports were positively correlated with penile amplitude.

In the preceding discussion we have referred to studies of the interaction between alcohol and expectation during varying blood alcohol levels. A statistically significant inverse linear relationship between penile tumescence and BAL was seen. The factor of expectation plays a far greater role when the dosage of alcohol is low and unvarying.

Marlatt and Rohsenow (1980) developed an experimental technique with alcohol using a balanced placebo design. Most investigations of the relationship between expectancy of alcohol's effect and its actual effect have used this "2 × 2 factorial design" since their report was published. In this type of experiment, subjects are placed in four different situations which can be characterized as follows: Expect Alcohol-Get No Alcohol; Expect Alcohol-Get Alcohol; Expect No Alcohol-Get No Alcohol; Expect No Alcohol-Get Alcohol. In their 1980 report, 1 part 80 proof vodka to 5 parts tonic water or plain tonic water were the beverages administered. This eliminated, to the authors' satisfaction, the chance that the actual beverage could be identified by the research subjects.

Earlier 2 × 2 designs had divided subjects into four situations but had not used a balanced placebo design. For example, Pliner and Cappell had reported on modifying the affective consequences of alcohol in solitary versus social situations. The social situation consisted of groups of three sitting on either side of a table drinking and not drinking. They were then asked to listen to a selection from a popular humorous recording. In the solitary situation, the subject was asked to supply captions for cartoons which had been supplied while not drinking and while intoxicated. The total sample consisted of 60 males and 60 females aged 18 to 30 recruited by a college newspaper ad. They were given a version of the Clyde mood scale to fill out during a pretest period. The drinking state was achieved by giving each subject a dose of 0.50 g/kg alcohol at a concentration of 25 percent.

Pliner and Cappell were satisfied that both of their predictions had been correct: (1) Subjects intoxicated in groups would describe their situation in affective terms whereas subjects intoxicated in a solitary situation described the same state in terms of physical conditions. (2) The manipulation of the social situation depended on the intoxicated state, that is, it had no effect in the placebo state. They conclude that alcohol and the environment "interact to determine the effectiveness of a drug" (Pliner and Cappell 1974). In *The Drinking Man*, Kalin (1972) had observed male subjects, some of whom had received alcohol, in the presence of an attractive female singer. There was no difference in the TAT response as a result of the singer's presence in the "dry" condition, but in the "wet" condition subjects responded with more sexual themes than subjects not exposed to her. Pliner and Cappell quoted this study in support of their own conclusion. In the Kalin study, amounts of alcohol and BALs were not documented.

Wilson has studied the interactions among alcohol, expectation and disinhibition with regard to social deviance very thoroughly. Wilson and Lawson found 40 undergraduate volunteers, all social drinkers, between the ages of 18 and 22. They were assigned randomly to one of two expectation conditions in which they were led to believe that the beverage they were drinking contained either vodka and tonic or tonic only. In each expectation condition, half of the subjects told to expect vodka and tonic got just tonic, and half that were told to expect tonic alone got vodka and tonic. The other two groups got what they were told to expect. Dosage of vodka was unvarying (either 0 or 1 part vodka to 5 parts tonic). The alcohol content of the alcohol-containing drinks was 0.5 g ethanol per kg body weight. After mixing the drink the subject completed a questionnaire indicating the effect he believed alcohol to have on sexual arousal in a natural setting. Breathalyzer tests were rigged so that the subject believed his drink to contain what he was told to expect. If subjects were told they were being given alcohol, their Breathalyzer readings read BAL 40 mg percent, regardless of what the actual drink contained. If subjects were told they were being given tonic only, their BAL indicators read 0 mg percent. Subjects were then given three TAT cards which were rated for responses manifesting sexual content. Subjects were also given a word association test that consisted of 50 words, 30 of which were double entendres. The remaining 20 words were neutral for sexual connotation. After completing the association test they were asked to speculate on what effect the beverage they were given would have on their sexual arousal when shown erotic films. Penile tumescence and penile diameter as well as skin temperature values associated with each change in penile diameter were recorded as the films were shown. In terms of pretest prediction, for the heterosexual film, 80 percent of the subjects in the "expect tonic-receive tonic" group and 90 percent in the other three groups predicted an increase in sexual arousal. For the homosexual film, 40 percent of the subjects in the two expect alcohol groups predicted an increase in arousal and only 10 and 20 percent respectively in the expect tonic groups predicted an increase. The results indicated no effect of alcohol on arousal. Those groups expecting alcohol manifested significantly greater sexual arousal to both homosexually and heterosexually erotic films regardless of the content of the drinks. No consistent results were documented in response to further measures of arousal, that is, TAT response, word association test, and skin response. Expectation about the effect of alcohol on arousal provided the subjects with permission to respond to homosexual films. I have one caveat about this finding: Prior to being asked to predict their responses to films, the subjects were told that their responses in the laboratory did not reflect their responses in a natural setting. They were also told that previous research had shown that heterosexual males often show some degree of arousal to homosexual stimuli. This suggests that the laboratory instructions enhanced expectation about the effect of alcohol on sexual response to homosexual stimuli. It is somewhat difficult to decipher whether expectation instructions provided by Wilson and Lawson or expectations about alcohol independent of the instructions played the more important role (Wilson and Lawson 1976).

In a further investigation, Lansky and Wilson used a balanced placebo design on 48 male social drinkers and concluded that "the belief that alcohol had been consumed increased penile tumescence to both heterosexual and homosexual stimuli, but only in subjects high in sex guilt" (Lansky and Wilson 1981: 35). There were 12 subjects per expectation group, that is, "per cell" (p. 37). In this experiment, consisting of respondents to a college newspaper ad who were aged 18 to 25, all were moderate drinkers, and considered themselves heterosexual and without sexual difficulty. They all drank an average of five cans of beer (60 oz.) per drinking occasion. The technique of manipulating belief about actual drink content was similar to the Wilson and Lawson experiment, with the further precaution that the volunteers gargled with Chloroseptic mouthwash to disguise the taste of their administered beverage. They were again told that it was natural to respond sexually to homosexual simulti in an experimental situation. Those drinks containing alcohol were pilot tested and found to produce BALs of 40 mg percent with a mixture of 1 part vodka to 4.17 parts tonic. Actual ethanol content of the drinks was 6 g ethanol per kg body weight. Three squirts of lime juice were added to all drinks to enhance the disguise of the contents. After a supervised 20-minute drinking period, subjects were placed in a dark room to watch slides and rate them on 7-point scales of arousal, obscenity, pleasure, eroticism, and interest.

Subjects were told they could view each slide as long as they wished and did not know that the length of time was being recorded. The student volunteers were viewed through a hidden television monitor. There were rigged Breathalyzer readings following the slide viewing. In a second phase, subjects heard heterosexual, homosexual, and nonsexual narratives through stereo headphones. Cognitive mathematical tasks were inserted between each story to counterbalance the order in which the students were presented with heterosexual and homosexual stimuli. Penile tumescence was recorded continuously while the narratives were heard. In a third phase, subjects were left with a slide memory booklet and asked to record whether they had definitely seen a particular slide, had probably seen it before, or had definitely not seen it before. Next, subjects filled out a sentence completion test of statements half of which had appeared in the narratives and half of which had not. The BALs for those subjects who had received alcohol were 20 mg percent at the beginning of the memory testing phase. After subjects had been assigned to expectation groups they were administered a Mosher F-C Inventory to assess sex guilt. A high and low sex guilt group was assigned to each Expectancy × Drink Content cell. The positive correlation between sex guilt and sexual responsiveness to homosexual stimuli in the expect alcohol groups is a further refinement of the earlier Wilson and Lawson experiment. Subjects had poorer memory for the slides they had viewed than for the narratives they had heard. Drink content had "a significantly deleterious effect on memory" (Lansky and Wilson 1981: 43). However, heterosexual slides were remembered most accurately, but the homosexual slides were remembered as having occurred more frequently than the heterosexual or nonsexual slides.

Lansky and Wilson state that, while this experiment supports the view of Lang et al. (1980) that subject variables, particularly degree of sexual guilt, are important modifiers of the alcohol expectancy effect, two qualifications must be made. First, only a low dose of alcohol was used, and it is not clear that the same expectancy effect would be observed in higher doses, and second, there were low levels of sexual guilt obtained for all subjects in this experiment. The finding that the taped narratives for which an expectancy effect was observed were rated as more stimulating suggested to Lansky and Wilson that occurrence of an alcohol expectancy effect depends in part on the potential of a stimulus for stimulation. There was no correlation between alcohol expectancy and slide viewing times.

In 1984 Wilson and Niaura published a paper that contradicted earlier results. Twenty-two male undergraduates aged 19 to 23 volunteered for experimental balanced placebo design conditions similar to the procedures of Wilson and Lawson (1976) and Lansky and Wilson (1981). Following administration of the beverage, subjects completed 20 minutes of the Minnesota Multiphasic Personality Inventory (MMPI) in order to distract them from noting internal sensations that might influence their expectations. Prior to participating in this study, subjects had taken part in a study that measured the effects of distraction on sexual arousal. They had been asked to perform different arithmetical tasks while listening to either erotic or neutral tapes presented simultaneously on a nonattended channel. All subjects had experienced this procedure prior to engaging in an experiment with the following instructions: They were asked to try as hard as they could to suppress sexual arousal while they listened to an audiotape of a man's voice describing his participation in foreplay, oral-genital contact, and coitus. Penile tumescence was measured continuously throughout the tape. Subjects who received alcohol-containing beverages had a BAL before the tape of 0.390 mg/dl following the drink administration and a BAL of 0.220 mg/dl after listening to the tape. Prior to hearing the tape, subjects completed a checklist of predictions about the effects of alcohol on their sexual arousal. After subjects were assigned to the four cells of the balanced placebo design, they were split on scores they had achieved on the Mosher Forced Choice Inventory, which was used to form high and low sexual guilt groups. Of the 22 subjects, 16 felt that moderate amounts of alcohol would increase their responsiveness but that large amounts would decrease it. Six subjects felt that alcohol would increase sexual responsiveness regardless of amount. Subjects were randomly distributed with regard to their predictions. A $2 \times 2 \times 2$ (drink content $\times$ expectancy $\times$ sexual guilt) analysis showed a significant effect of drink content on latency to onset of penile tumescence. No other significant effects of expectancy or sexual guilt on penile tumescence were found. This is the first report in which a low and fixed dose of alcohol in a balanced placebo design experiment demonstrated a physiological effect on penile tumescence latency regardless of expectation of sexual guilt (Wilson and Niaura 1984).

Effect of BAL on Ejaculatory Response

Malatesta et al. (1979) selected 24 adult, nonalcoholic heterosexual, healthy male volunteers, aged 22 to 34, and measured their ejaculatory responses with varying doses of alcohol which were designed to achieve four different BAL levels. Because Masters and Johnson had reported the likelihood of intersubject differences (Masters and Johnson 1966), counterbalancing of experimental sessions and videotape presentations was part of the design framework in an effort to control for habituation and/or sequence effects. Latency of ejaculation was measured with EMG recordings of decreases in genital muscle activity at the beginning of orgasm and by providing the research participant with a response button connected to the polygraph with which the participant could signal the onset of orgasm. Raw heart rate was measured with two electrode discs attached to the left arm and leg and connected to the polygraph. Each participant took part in five sessions: a desensitization session and four experimental sessions. Each session took place at 48-hour intervals and was approximately 2 hours long. Prior to each session, each participant refrained from sex for 24 hours and from food for 4 hours. One of four blood alcohol concentrations was sustained per session as follows: 0.0 percent, 0.03 percent, 0.06 percent, and 0.09 percent. After reaching the desired BAC, the subject listened to an instrumental soundtrack while baseline EMG genital muscle recordings and heart rate were obtained. Following this, subjects saw one of four sexually explicit videotapes each lasting 16 minutes while asked to masturbate to orgasm and ejaculation. Ten of the subjects did not attain orgasm during the 16-minute session for the two higher BACs. Ejaculation latency scores under the no-alcohol placebo condition were much shorter than for those obtained at 0.06 and 0.09 percent but not for 0.03 percent. Malatesta et al. (1979) conclude that "increasing levels of alcohol intoxication produce a significant degradation in male masturbatory effectiveness." They observed that the increased latency effect of alcohol was complemented further by various subjective criteria, that is, decreased sexual arousal, decreased sexual pleasure, decreased intensity of orgasm, and reported difficulty in attaining orgasm. This finding was felt to have important therapeutic implications in a twofold way: First, knowledge of this effect could be used to allay anxiety by correcting a mislabeled dysfunctional heterosexual experience; and second, as a beneficial consequence, to delay ejaculation purposely in order to produce a prolongation of intercourse which both partners prefer. This is the only published study of which I am aware in which physiological measurements were used to determine the effect of alcohol on ejaculatory response specifically.

Indirect Experimental Measures of the Effect of Alcohol on Sexual Responsiveness of Male Social Drinkers

Clark (1952) and Clark and Sensibar (1955) measured TAT scores among college student volunteers in drinking and nondrinking situations. In both investigations it was concluded that under normal conditions sexual arousal evokes guilt sufficient to inhibit the expression of sex. Alcohol was said to reduce the guilt over arousal enough to permit the expression of sex accompanied by a resulting increase in expressed guilt. Experimental groups were prestimulated by slides of nude women, or the presence of an attractive female. Control groups were not prestimulated. Both were exposed to drinking or nondrinking situations. McClelland et al. (1972) reported on 10 years of research into the role of alcohol in human life, with sexuality and interest in participating in sexual acts among the variables examined. Extensive use was made of the TAT. Most subjects were male college students. Sexual themes expressed in projective tests were thought to indicate need for power. A year prior to the publication of *The Drinking Man* (McClelland et al. 1972), Carpenter and Armenti (1971) expressed serious methodological reservations about investigations that utilized these tests as the primary basis for formulating conclusions. One criticism was that only male subjects were used. In addition, the criteria for choosing amounts of alcohol for subjects to drink was not defined, and BACs, when reported, were sometimes much higher than would be expected in normal human drinking situations. Furthermore, the meaning of the sexual content on the TAT was unclear in terms of the experimental provocations and in the implications of the findings for behavior.

Lang et al. (1980) employed the balanced placebo design with 72 male undergraduates who were selected on the basis of their low, moderate, and high scores on the Sex Guilt subscale of the Mosher Forced-Choice Guilt Inventory. The amount of alcohol given in the alcohol-receiving cells produced a BAL between 30 and 40 mg/100 ml. All subjects viewed color slides selected to elicit pornographic rating responses. Viewing times increased as a positive linear function of the pornographic content of the slides. Cards with the most explicit pornographic content were viewed longer than cards with less explicit or no pornographic content. The more pornographic the card, the longer the card was viewed. In the high sex guilt groups, those who were instructed to expect alcohol viewed the slides for a significantly longer period than those who were instructed to expect tonic. Only the high guilt scorers who were told to expect tonic did not increase their viewing times. Subjects also rated slides as more stimulating if they had been instructed to expect alcohol irrespective of drink content. Wilson refers to Lansky's unpublished doctoral dissertation in which he followed almost the same procedure as Lang et al. with some differences. Lansky's slides showed homosexual and nonsexual scenes as well as heterosexual content. The BAL was slightly higher and, in addition, subjects were not assigned to groups on the basis of their sex guilt scores. Lang's findings were not replicated. Expectation of drink content did not affect slide viewing times. The only variable that affected viewing time was the content; subjects looked at heterosexual slides longer than other slides (Wilson 1981).

Ability to delay gratification and its relationship to alcohol consumption has also been studied. Using a balanced placebo design and a fixed low BAL, subjects were given a choice after consuming their drinks and watching 45 seconds of an erotic film. They were told that the longer they waited to see the film, the more of the film they could see. Subjects who believed that they consumed alcohol waited significantly longer than those who believed they had consumed tonic regardless of actual drink content. In addition, subjects who thought they had been drinking reported more sexual thoughts as well as decreased embarassment and increased pleasure during the delay phase. High sex guilt scorers displayed a significantly shorter delay time than lower sex guilt scorers, but this was not related to their alcohol consumption expectation instructions as it had been in the Lang study (Abrams and Wilson, unpublished study cited in Wilson, 1981).

SUMMARY

Until recently, most careful research using the balanced placebo design to measure expectation yielded results strongly in support of the hypothesis that expectation of alcohol's effect influences behavior independently of drink content when low doses of alcohol are used. Wilson and Niaura's 1984 paper measuring penile tumescence response to expectancy contradicts this, as does Lansky's replication of Lang's experimental conditions using slightly higher doses of alcohol (Wilson 1981: 26-27). In the Wilson and Niaura paper, alcohol played a greater role than expectation on physiological responsiveness and, in Lansky's study, as cited by Wilson, slide content played a larger role than either expectation or alcohol on slide viewing time.

The balanced placebo design experiments and physiological measurements of sexual responsiveness using calculated doses of alcohol have combined to provide better research methodology. We must await further investigation before reaching definitive conclusions about the interrelationship betwen drink content and expectation. At higher doses of alcohol, the negative physiological and hormonal effects on the sexual response of nonalcoholic social drinkers are much more conclusive.

REFERENCES

Abel, E. L. 1985. *Psychoactive Drugs and Sex* (New York: Plenum Press).

Abrams, D. B., and G. T. Wilson. 1981. "The Effects of Alcohol and Expectations of Drinking on Delay of Gratification." Cited in Wilson, 1981: 28-29.

Amir, M. 1967. "Alcohol and Forcible Rape." *Br. J. Addict.* 62:219-32.

Athanasiou, R., P. Shaver, and C. Tavris. 1970. "Sex." *Psychol. Today* 4:37-52.

Beigel, H. 1967. "Illegitimacy." In *Encyclopaedia of Sexual Behavior,* edited by A. Ellis and A. Abarbanel (New York: Hawthorn Books), pp. 563-772.

Briddell, D. W., and G. T. Wilson. 1976. "The Effects of Alcohol and Expectancy Set on Male Sexual Arousal." *J. Abnorm. Psychol.* 85: 225-34.

Carpenter, A., and N. P. Armenti. 1971. "Some Effects of Ethanol on Human Sexual and Aggressive Behavior." In *The Biology of Alcoholism,* edited by B. Kissin and H. Begleiter (New York: Plenum Press), pp. 509-43.

Cicero, T. J. 1980. "Common Mechanisms Underlying the Effects of Ethanol and the Narcotics on Neuroendocrine Function." In *Advances in Substance Abuse,* Vol. 1, edited by N. K. Mello (Greenwich, CT: JAI Press), pp. 201-54.

———. 1982. "Alcohol-Induced Deficits in the Hypothalamic-Pituitary-Luteinizing Hormone Axis in the Male." *Alcoholism: Clin. Exptl. Res.* 6, no. 2:207-12.

Cicero, T. J., D. Bernstein, and T. M. Badger. 1978. "Effects of Acute Alcohol Administration on Reproductive Endocrinology in the Male Rat." *Alcoholism: Clin. Exptl. Res.* 2:249-54.

Clark, R. A. 1952. "The Projective Measurement of Experimentally Induced Levels of Sexual Motivation." *J. Exptl. Psychol.* 44:391-99.

Clark, R. A., and M. R. Sensibar. 1955. "The Relationship Between Symbolic and Manifest Projections of Sexuality with Some Incidental Correlates." *J. Abnorm. Psychol.* 50:327-34.

Farkas, G. M., and R. C. Rosen. 1976. "Effect of Alcohol on Elicited Male Sexual Response." *J. Stud. Alcohol* 37, no. 3:265-72.

Gallup, G. 1986. "Women: A Powerful Force for Moderation." *Alcoholism Addict.* (November-December):13.

Gebhard, P. H., J. H. Gagnon, W. B. Pomeroy, and C. V. Christenson, eds. 1965. *Sex Offenders: An Analysis of Types* (New York: Harper & Row and Paul B. Hoeber Medical Books).

Goodwin, D. 1976. *Is Alcoholism Hereditary?* (New York: Oxford University Press).

Goodwin, D. W., J. B. Crane, and S. B. Guze. 1971. "Felons Who Drink: An 8-Year Follow-up." *Q. J. Studies Alcohol* 32:136-47.

Gordon, G. G., K. Altman, A. L. Southren, E. Rubin, and C. S. Lieber. 1976. "Effect of Alcohol Administration on Sex-Hormone Metabolism in Normal Men." *N. Engl. J. Med.* 295, no. 15:793-97.

Johnson, H. J. 1974. *Executive Life Styles: A Life Extension Report on Alcohol, Sex and Health* (New York: Thomas Y. Crowell, Company).

Kalin, R. 1972. "Social Drinking in Different Settings." In *The Drinking Man,* edited by D. C. McClelland, W. N. Davis, R. Kalin, and E. Wanner (New York: The Free Press), pp. 21-44.

Kaplan, H. 1974. *The New Sex Therapy* (New York: Brunner/Mazel in cooperation with Times Books) pp. 88-89, 98.

———. 1979. *The New Sex Therapy, Vol. 2: Disorders of Sexual Desire* (New York: Brunner/Mazel), Appendix, Table 1, p. 1.

Knight, R. P. 1937. "The Psychodynamics of Chronic Alcoholism." *J. Nerv. Ment. Dis.* 86:538-48.

Lang, A. R., D. J. Goekner, V. J. Adesso, and G. A. Marlatt. 1975. "Effects of Alcohol on Aggression in Male Social Drinkers." *J. Abnorm. Psychol.* 84, no. 5:508-18.

Lang, A. R., J. Searles, R. Lauerman, and V. Adesso. 1980. "Expectancy, Alcohol and Sex Guilt as Determinants of Interest in and Reaction to Sexual Stimuli." *J. Abnorm. Psychol.* 89:644-53.

Lansky, D. 1980. "Alcohol, Expectations, and Sexual Arousal: An Information Processing Analysis." Doctoral diss., Rutgers University, 1980. Cited in Wilson, 1981.

Lansky, D., and G. T. Wilson. 1981. "Alcohol, Expectations, and Sexual Arousal in Males: An Information Processing Analysis." *J. Abnorm. Psychol.* 90, no. 1:35-45.

Malatesta, V. J., R. H. Pollack, W. A. Wilbanks, and H. E. Adams. 1979. "Alcohol Effects on the Orgasmic-Ejaculatory Response in Human Males," *J. Sex Res.* 15, no. 2:101-7.

Marlatt, G. A., and D. J. Rohsenow. 1980. "Cognitive Processes in Alcohol Use: Expectancy and the Balanced Placebo Design," In *Advances in Substance Abuse,* vol. 1, edited by N. K. Mello (Greenwich, CT: JAI Press), pp. 159-99.

Masters, W., and V. Johnson. 1966. *Human Sexual Response* (Boston, MA: Little, Brown and Company), pp. 267-68.

______. 1970. *Human Sexual Inadequacy* (Boston, MA: Little, Brown and Company), pp. 163-68.

McClelland, D. C., W. N. Davis, R. Kalin, and E. Wanner, eds. 1972. *The Drinking Man* (New York: The Free Press).

Pliner, P., and H. Cappell. 1974. "Modification of Affective Consequences of Alcohol: A Comparison of Social and Solitary Drinking." In *J. Abnorm. Psychol.* 3, no. 4:418-25.

Rada, R. T. 1975. "Alcohol and Rape." *Med. Aspects Hum. Sex.* 9:48-65.

______. 1975. "Alcoholism and Forcible Rape." *Am. J. Psychiatr.* 132: 444-46.

Ratliff, K. G., and B. R. Burkhart. 1984. "Sex Differences in Motivations for and Effects of Drinking Among College Students." *J. Stud. Alcohol* 45, no. 1:26-32.

Rockwell, K., E. Ellenwood, C. Kantor, W. Maack, and J. Schrumpf. 1973. "Drugs and Sex: Scene of Ambivalence." *College Health* 21: 483-88.

Rubin, E., C. S. Lieber, K. Altman, G. Gordon, and H. Southren. 1976. "Prolonged Ethanol Consumption Increases Testosterone Metabolism in the Liver." *Science* 191:563-64.

Rubin, H. B., and D. E. Henson. 1976. "Effects of Alcohol on Male Sexual Responding." *Psychopharmacology* 47:123-34.

Van Thiel, D., and R. Lester. 1974. "Sex and Alcohol." *N. Engl. J. Med.* 291:252-53.

Weitzman, E. D., R. M. Boyar, S. Kapen, et al. 1975. "The Relationship of Sleep and Sleep Stages to Neuroendocrine Secretion and Biological Rhythms in Man." *Recent Prog. Horm. Res.* 31:399-446.

Wilson, G. T. 1977. "Alcohol and Human Sexual Behavior." *Behav. Res. Ther.* 15:239-52.

———. 1981. "The Effects of Alcohol on Human Sexual Behavior." In *Advances in Substance Abuse,* vol. 2 (Greenwich, CT: JAI Press), pp. 1-40.

Wilson, G. T., and D. M. Lawson. 1976. "Expectancies, Alcohol, and Sexual Arousal in Male Social Drinkers." *J. Abnorm. Psychol.* 85, no. 6:587-94.

Wilson, G. T., and R. Niaura. 1984. "Alcohol and the Disinhibition of Sexual Responsiveness." *J. Stud. Alcohol* 45, no. 3:219-24.

Ylikahri, R., M. Huttunen, M. Harkonen, and H. Adlercreutz. 1974. "Hangover and Testosterone." *Br. Med. J.* 2:445.

Ylikahri, R., M. Huttunen, M. Harkonen, U. Seuderling, S. Onikki, S. L. Kardnen, and H. Adlercreutz. 1974. "Low Plasma Testosterone Values in Men During Hangover." *J. Steroid Biochem.* 5:655-58.

2

Sexual Response in Male Alcoholics

Chronic alcohol abuse produces hormonal, physiological, and psychosocial consequences, all of which affect sexuality adversely.

Because alcoholism and sexuality had been largely neglected as proper fields for research concentration until the middle 1960s, most of the earlier papers are anecdotal and appear to be biased in favor of prevailing cultural impressions and psychoanalytic theories about the etiology of alcoholism. Additional factors hampering the development of knowledge had been poor research methodology and a professional separation between the subspecialities of alcoholism and human sexuality. It is only in the 1980s that the two areas have overlapped as subjects of importance for clinicians and researchers. Even now specialists in substance abuse know little about human sexuality, and sexologists rarely study the impact of substance abuse on their patients.

Endocrinologists gathered the first solid data about the effects of alcohol over time on the hypothalamic-pituitary-gonadal axis and the resultant sexual consequences. Personality changes during intoxication have been investigated with reference to marital adjustment, the adaptation of alcoholic homosexuals, the sexual adaptation of single, heterosexual male alcoholics, and the incidence of sexual crimes and sexual deviance.

Rehabilitated alcoholics deal frequently with problems surrounding sexual adaptation in a sober state, and the available clinical data on this will also be discussed in this chapter.

Finally, experimental investigations involving the separate effects of alcohol and expectation on penile tumescence in chronic alcoholics will be described.

CLINICAL OBSERVATIONS AND CORRELATIONAL INVESTIGATIONS

Hormonal

There is general agreement that testosterone levels in chronic alcoholics are dramatically lower than in controls (Abel 1985; Van Thiel and Gavaler 1985; Cicero 1980; Chiao and Van Thiel 1983; Scheig 1975; Ellingboe and Varinelli 1979; Gordon, Southren, and Lieber 1978, 1979). Controversy reigns over how this effect is produced.

The feminization effect produced by advanced alcoholic liver disease is established. It is common for men with liver disease to experience a decrease in chest, axillary, and pubic hair and the development of a female escutcheon. Their appearance is unattractive and this in itself would tend to decrease sexual intimacy (Scheig 1975). A person with ascites may find it difficult to find a comfortable position for intercourse, since the abdomen may be blown up to a size resembling advanced pregnancy (Scheig 1975). Van Thiel notes that not only is there a depletion of testosterone in males with chronic liver disease, but there is also hyperestrogenization. However, the magnitude of increase in levels of plasma estrone, estradiol, and prolactin does not necessarily correlate with overt changes in appearance (Van Thiel 1977). The damaged liver allows increased hepatic release of the weak androgen, androstenedione, to peripheral sites where it is converted to estrone (Southren et al. 1973; Gordon et al. 1975). This is associated with weak hepatic estrone uptake (summarized by Van Thiel, 1977). There is a direct toxic effect of alcohol on the gonads even in the absence of liver disease (Gordon, Southren, and Lieber, 1979; Van Thiel 1977; Lester, Eagon, and Van Thiel 1979; Mendelson and Mello 1979; Cicero 1980).

Controversy exists over whether the hypothalamus and pituitary are affected by alcohol and thus contribute to the depletion of testosterone and testicular atrophy. *In vitro* gonadatropin (specifically, LH) binding to Leydig cell receptors in the testes is reduced by alcohol. It is not clear that this also occurs *in vivo* because the levels of alcohol needed to produce this effect *in vitro* are quite high (Chiao and Van Thiel 1983). The *in vitro* binding loss is due to destruction of surface Leydig cell gonadatropin receptors (Bhalla, Chen, and Granaprakasam 1979). There is also a loss of Leydig cell cyclic AMP *in vitro* but again, there is no definitive evidence that this occurs *in vivo* (Rajan et al. 1982). Oxidation of ethanol by alcohol dehydrogenase to acetaldehyde and oxidation of acetaldehyde by acetaldehyde dehydrogenase to acetate requires a reduction of Nicotinamide Adenine Dinucleotide from its oxidized state, NAD, to its reduced state, NADH, in order to occur. As a result, the NAD/NADH ratio of the cell is reduced. Since NAD is important in testicular steriodogenesis, many investigators have hypothesized that the reduction of NAD in the Leydig cells of alcoholics is responsible for the adverse effect of alcohol on testosterone production (Van Thiel et al. 1981; Ellingboe and Varinelli 1979; Van Thiel and Lester 1974, 1976; Gordon et al. 1980). Data has accumulated showing that both ethanol and acetaldehyde are capable of inhibiting several of the microsomal enzymes involved in steriodogenesis (Johnston et al. 1981; Cicero et al. 1980; Chiao et al. 1981). Acetaldehyde can inhibit 17-alpha-hydroxyprogesterone aldolase, which further limits testosterone biosynthesis (Johnston et al. 1981).

Outside the Leydig cells, there are two mechanisms that have been postulated to interfere with testosterone production. In the liver, alcohol enhances metabolism of testosterone because it induces alpha-5-reductase and aromatase activity. Alpha-5-reductase is the enzyme involved in the first step of testosterone breakdown to dihydrotestosterone; aromatase completes the conversion of testosterone to estrogens (Gordon et al. 1979b; Vittek et al. 1981; Rubin et al. 1976; Gordon, Southren, Vittek and Lieber 1979a).

There is evidence that, after prolonged exposure to ethanol, alpha reductase is reduced, which leaves the mechanism for extragonadal testicular failure uncertain (Chiao and Van Thiel 1983: 132).

Some data suggests that alcoholic men have increased response to normal levels of estrogen. Either there are more estrogen receptors available in these men or they have a reduced capacity to prevent estrogen uptake by estrogen receptors. Both situations have been reported in the liver (Eagon et al. 1981).

Further investigation is necessary to determine whether estrogen increases because one or both of these two mechanisms take place in the hypothalamus and pituitary. Estrogens and androgens inhibit LH secretion which, in turn, inhibits Leydig cell function. It is possible, therefore, as Chiao and Van Thiel (1983: 133) suggest, that the increased estrogenic activity decreases Leydig cell steroidogenesis. They suggest also that ethanol produces a resultant decrease in LH secretion by the pituitary and luteinizing hormone releasing hormone (LHRH, also referred to as LRF, or releasing factor) from the hypothalamus.

Cicero's (1980) data on rats indicates simultaneous decrease in LH and testosterone as a result of ethanol administration. In humans who have imbibed alcohol LH is inconsistently low. Cicero suggests that since LH normally increases as a result of testosterone decrease in the circulation, the failure of LH to rise supports the theory of a direct toxic effect of alcohol on the pituitary and/or hypothalamus.

Lemere and Smith believe that impotence after years of sobriety is neither hormonal nor psychological but due to destruction by alcohol of the reflex arc involved with erection (Lemere and Smith 1973: 212). This arc is said to include "(1) the cerebral cortex, from which sexual thoughts arise, (2) the anterior portion of the temporal lobe, which determines intensity of libido, (3) perhaps the hypothalamus, (4) the spinal cord reflex centers for erection, and (5) the peripheral nerves that convey sensory and vasomotor impulses to and from the genital organs. The mechanism for this might be compared to the diminution of sexual ability complicating the generalized nervous system damage caused by uncontrolled diabetes." They consider treatment ineffective "except to warn heavy drinkers . . . to stop drinking in the hope that sobriety and time will restore their sexual vigor" (p. 213).

Sexual Desire in Male Alcoholics

Levine (1953) scrutinized the records of all alcoholics who had received psychotherapy in a state-run outpatient clinic. He selected 79 charts for completeness. The majority of this mixed group had sexual intercourse infrequently. Of 63 men, 44 did not have sexual intercourse more often than once every three months. In therapy interviews, they expressed indifference or complete lack of interest in sex. Twelve of the 44 had intercourse only once or twice a year.

Two of these men "were known to be overt homosexuals." The two active homosexuals said that they could engage in sex with male partners only when drunk. Nineteen of the 63 reported sexual intercourse once or twice a week. Three men emphasized their heterosexual interest; however, one of these had erectile dysfunction. The second had frequent extramarital relations but experienced sexual dysfunction with his wife, and the third was thought to use sex as reassurance of his wife's interest in him.

Levine concludes that the effect of alcohol on desire is frequently in the direction of diminished sexual interest and that when alcohol is accompanied by increased sexual activity, there is impairment in performance. The increased demand for sex in these latter cases may be motivated by the need to be secure about masculinity, rather than by heightened libido. However, he offers a psychological explanation for this rather than a physiological one. He reports that nearly 75 percent of the men had a strongly dominant mother and a weak, distant father. Several men remained bachelors and lived with their mothers or married much older women. The men often expressed overt anger toward their fathers but never toward their mothers, and there was no male figure with whom they could identify. Levine says that these findings are consistent with the psychoanalytic hypothesis of Karl Abraham that the alcoholic has a basic homosexual problem.

Jensen (1979) studied several variables with respect to sexuality gathered from male alcoholics. Information was obtained from 100 men aged 30 to 45. Sixty-three percent of the men complained of sexual dysfunction, particularly erectile dysfunction and diminished libido. Jensen concluded that problems originated in psychological and interpersonal realms and based this on a lack of correlation between duration of alcoholism and sexual difficulty. He said that low self-esteem, chronic fatigue, few interpersonal contacts, abrupt change from drinking to treatment and abstinence, changes in the power balance with abstinence, a "loser" socioeconomic status, and finally, drugs, alcoholic dementia, and neuropathy were the factors involved. In the absence of physiological factors, sex therapy for couples was advised. Hormonal factors were never mentioned and any physical factors were considered neurogenic in origin.

No synchrony exists between the conclusions reached by Levine and Jensen and the findings of endocrinologists. This tunnel-vision compartmentalization illustrates one of the major obstacles on the road to a coherent understanding of alcohol's effect on human sexuality. Psychiatrists and psychologists seldom familiarize themselves with developments in other biological sciences, and therefore these findings have only recently begun to be utilized in counseling alcoholic patients with sexual problems. Levine's article antedates almost all of the endocrinologists' work. It is nevertheless striking that he doesn't consider neurophysiological factors at all in attributing causes for diminished sexual desire. Jensen, writing in 1979, makes only a passing allusion to "neuropathy" (Jensen 1979: 34).

In his recent treatment-oriented monograph, Forrest (1983: 17) asserts that alcoholism is an acting-out to repair the injury caused by the absence of "an intensely loving anxiety-free fusion with the mother object." Prior to the onset of alcoholism, the alcoholic is thought to have sustained severe and chronic narcissistic injury, which could render the male phobic about female genitals as well as anxious and embarrassed about sexual performance. Low sexual desire is thought to be a defense against all of the above. Forrest recommends teaching of social skills and assertiveness training as well as relaxation techniques, and replacement of unpleasant heterosexual imagery with pleasant associations. Hormonal treatment is suggested as a last resort.

Whalley's (1978) study of the sexual adjustment of male alcoholics compared the sexual attitudes of 50 hospitalized male alcoholics with a matched control sample from the general population. He found no appreciable differences in sexual attitudes between the two groups. Age at first intercourse was lower among alcoholics and Whalley thinks that this was due to a higher degree of impulsivity and recklessness. He states that there is "no support" for the view that alcoholics have low sexual interest, incomplete masculine identification, or tend to marry older women. Alcoholic subjects did describe less sexual satisfaction, attributed by Whalley to "greater interest in sex, loss of erectile potency and lack of a sexual partner." Penick, Powell, and Read (1984) hypothesized that the proportion of alcoholic men in their sample who had feminine role orientation had developed it in reaction to a chronic illness (i.e., alcoholism). In contrast, Douglas and Nutter (1986), using masculinity and femininity pretreatment and post-treatment scales with 66 men and 65 women, found that men consistently scored in the "passive-feminine" range.

Alcoholic men were atypical of men in the general population. Womens' sex-role orientation closely matched that of nonalcoholic women. They concluded that this type of sex-role orientation preceded the onset of the addiction. One caveat that must be stated in response to this study is that scales of masculinity and femininity are designed in accordance with arbitrary designations of what is masculine or feminine. These determinations are influenced by the cultural stereotypes prevailing at the time the scales were developed, and may or may not be true measures of sexual orientation. Mandell and Miller (1983) found high rates of sexual dysfunction in their sample of 44 outpatients in a county alcoholism program. Fifty-three percent were still drinking actively. Quantity of alcohol consumed, duration of drinking from onset of regular drinking to the present time, and frequency of drinking affected sexual function. During heavy drinking, 59 percent experienced erectile dysfunction and 48 percent suffered from ejaculatory incompetence. A large majority (84.4 percent) had at least one kind of sexual dysfunction. If drinking decreased, older men with histories of fewer problems prior to onset of drinking had improvement in sexual functioning. Younger men in whom sexual dysfunction was high prior to drinking did not improve with reduction of alcohol consumption. Men who drank 28 oz. or more of alcohol per day were most likely to experience ejaculatory retardation with full erection despite stimulation. In these instances there was some improvement with decline in drinking, but the improvement did not reach statistical significance.

One would think that if chronic alcoholism decreases sexual desire, then hormone replacement is an option. Van Thiel and Lester (1976) consider hormonal replacement therapy a Pandora's box. They caution that administration of testosterone might increase facial hair and potency but could further impair spermatogenesis and would not affect feminization due to increased estrogen.

They found that clomiphene produces a transient effect by interrupting steroid feedback control of the hypothalamus and thus increasing plasma LH concentrations. But clomiphene is weakly estrogenic and might adversely affect patients who already show signs of hyperestrogenization. Little is known about prolonged effects.

Substance abuse therapists stress that marital therapy, particularly for sexual issues, should not be addressed until abstinence from alcohol has been established for at least six months. This is because it requires intense concentration for the thinking habits necessary to maintain abstinence from alcohol to become second nature (Forrest 1983; Powell 1984; Shirley and Shirley 1981).

Case Report

T.J., aged 56, was hospitalized at Silver Hill Foundation because of severe physiological dependence on alcohol. Prior to admission, he abstained from alcohol only during his 8-hour shift at a scientific instruments firm. At all other times he drank continuously while awake. He had become estranged from his wife because he was often sleepy, or morose and noncommunicative. His self-esteem was low due to his readily acknowledged inability to stop drinking. He was isolated from family members and friends. His work performance was marginal and he was often absent or late. Before his drinking had interfered with his life, he reported having had a satisfying sexual relationship with intercourse at least twice a week. In his early years of heavy drinking he experienced full penile tumescence and ejaculation when masturbating. Such occasions became progressively rare due to decreased libido. His wife had rejected him sexually because he reeked of alcohol. After a while he stopped making sexual advances to her and there had been no attempt at sexual intercourse for over 10 years. He had no extramarital affairs because he preferred to come home from work, go to the cellar (so that he wouldn't be nagged about drinking), and drink.

He had not thought of himself in a sexual role for years. "I think that part of my life is just over. I'll be lucky if my wife even talks to me, and I don't think I care much about sex anymore anyway."

Mrs. J. refused to be involved in conjoint sessions with her husband, his alcoholism counselor, and myself. According to her husband she thought his drinking was his problem and not her responsibility. This, while true, gave her no forum to air her own pain and resentment. It gave Mr. and Mrs. J. no opportunity to begin repairing their relationship.

When T. left the hospital he had become strongly motivated to improve the quality of his life in nonsexual areas. He remained alcohol-free, attended AA enthusiastically on a daily basis, and developed close friendships in that fellowship. His work improved and he was promoted.

His wife maintained an icy silence for several months. When she became secure about T.'s intention to stay sober, she began conversing with him and, very gradually, they began going to movies and seeing friends and relatives together. They never revived their sexual relationship, but T.J. was content with his situation.

This case was summarized to illustrate absent sexual desire in a chronic alcoholic male. Hormone levels were not determined, so we cannot be sure that this patient's decreased libido was due to any hormone deficiency. T.J.'s sexual life seemd quite normal prior to the onset of his excessive drinking pattern. I don't believe that the change in his sexual adaptation can be attributed to intrapsychic conflicts that preceded his addiction. We never had the opportunity to speak to Mrs. J. Since involvement of family members in treatment is our usual practice, Mrs. J.'s avoidance of us in itself suggests intense hostility toward her husband. We learned only about the pre-morbid and post-morbid psychosexual adjustment of Mr. J. and can only speculate about whether Mrs. J.'s lack of interest in sexual activity with her husband contributed to their asexual relationship after his recovery. We know that Mr. J. was interested in sex before he became ill, but we don't know if Mrs. J. were merely compliant or actually desired intercourse. In any event, since the situation was not causing Mr. J. any distress, we did not pursue a recommendation of sexual therapy for the couple. At least Mr. and Mrs. J. were on speaking terms, and we didn't want to upset the balance.

Incidence of Sex Crimes in Male Alcoholics

Rape

As indicated in the last chapter, there is disagreement about alcohol's role in the incidence of rape. Amir cited drinking in the offender in 24 percent of 646 cases of forcible rape, 3 percent of offenders only, and 21 percent of cases in which both the victim and the offender had been drinking (Amir 1967). Tinklenberg and Woodrow (1974) were also unimpressed with the association between intoxication and sexual offenses.

Rada (1975) found a 50 percent correlation between drinking and forcible rape in data collected from detailed autobiographies of 77 convicted rapists. Thirty-five percent of the rapists who were drinking were alcoholics. Rada stresses the importance of follow-up treatment for the alcoholic sexual offender, which would address alcoholism as well as impaired sexual adjustment. Gagnon (1977: 310-11), studying imprisoned rapists, concluded that they, unlike those who have enough social skill to rape without being arrested, are socially incompetent. He thinks that their poor judgment may have further deteriorated with intoxication at the time of the crime, but it is not clear how many imprisoned rapists are alcoholics.

Mendelson and Mello (1974) carried out a study with sober alcoholics who were residents of a correctional and rehabilitation facility. Three categories of violent behavior were established according to degree of violence. Testosterone levels were correlated with histories of violent behavior and no clear association could be made. This contrasted with findings of other investigators who found direct correlations between testosterone levels and violence (Persky, Smith, and Basu 1971; Rose, Holady, and Bernstein 1971; Rose, Borden, and Bernstein 1972; Kreuz and Rose 1972). The implication of this dissociation between testosterone level and aggression is that the drop in testosterone found to occur after alcohol ingestion may have no moderating influence on aggressive impulses. If alcohol ingestion increases the incidence of violent crimes, it is apparently not caused by hormonal changes. Rada, Laws, and Kellner (1976) attempted to correlate plasma testosterone levels in rapists and child molesters who completed the Michigan Alcoholism Screening Test as well as psychometric hostility assessments. The group judged to be most hostile were alcoholic rapists. They had a significantly higher mean plasma testosterone level than nonalcoholic rapists.

A more recent study found a high correlation between the incidence of rape and occurrence of drinking among the perpetrators (Filmore 1985; Gallant 1986).

While some investigators have concluded that alcohol consumption plays a significant role in the perpetration of rape, others are unconvinced about the presence of a correlation. Whether alcohol serves merely as an excuse for rape, or actually facilitates rape by impairing judgment in men who would not have been rapists if they had not been drunk, is a question that remains unanswered. Lack of clarity also persists about the respective influences of alcohol and testosterone levels on violent behavior.

Incest

Just as with rape, there is controversy over the degree to which alcoholism correlates with the rate of incest. Scott (1977) believed that the fathers who committed incest in his group of cases claimed alcoholic blackouts, but the ingestion of alcohol was planned as an excuse for the incestuous activity. Virkkunen (1974) studied 45 cases of incest in which 22 cases suggested alcoholism in the offender as determined by daily drinking over long periods of the day for several years. The group who had been designated alcoholics were more likely to have histories of violent criminal offenses. They also had been more aggressive at home prior to the onset of the incest.

The spouse had rejected the offender sexually in the cases in which alcoholism had been a factor. The reasons for this were disgust with the alcohol abuse, large families, and poor living conditions. In more than half of both groups, actual intercourse had taken place. The alcoholic father tended to be under the influence of alcohol at least at the beginning of the sexual relationship. Westermeyer (1978) says that alcohol and drug abuse occur in cases of incest but are not universal.

Cavallin (1966) reported on 12 cases of incest among 381 felons. Four of these men drank excessively. A higher incidence of alcoholism was found in Phillip's (1966) study of 182 cases of incestuous fathers in which 50 percent were alcoholic. Meiselman (1978) found an incidence of alcoholism in 20 percent of cases involving father-daughter incest. Daughters would explain the incest as a function of their father's alcoholism.

Some investigators point out that men are more frequent victims of incest than previously estimated (Westermeyer 1978; Finkelhor 1980). Awad (1976) reported a case of father-son incest in which the father's drinking produced a breakdown of his social or "ego" controls during the incidents. The husband's abstinence was a primary goal of conjoint marital therapy. Reynolds (1986) cites an incidence of paternal alcoholism in 60 percent of her sexually abused clients at the Institute Against Social Violence. The ratios of female to male perpetrators and victims are not stated. Liles and Childs

(1986) have found similarities in the dynamics of families in which incest or alcohol abuse has occurred. Liles surveyed 264 therapists treating father-daughter incest cases in specialized sexual abuse treatment programs in the United States. Alcohol was used by the perpetrators as a disinhibitor "to make it easier to commit the molestations." Although Liles and Childs note that denial, minimalization, and rationalization typify families in which alcoholism and/or incest exists, they do not make the case that incestuous behavior is caused by the alcoholism.

Pedophilia

There is polarized opinion about the correlation between drinking and child molesting. Conclusions range from a disproportionately high association with alcoholim (Aarens et al. 1977; Rada 1976) to the concept of alcoholism as a vehicle for denying deviance (McCaghy 1968; Swanson 1968). Those who see child molestation and incest as behavior occurring in the course of an alcoholic blackout recommend that treatment should focus on substance abuse rehabilitation. Alcoholics can save face if they can blame child abuse on their alcoholism. (A blackout is defined here as a state in which the perpetrator is under the influence of alcohol and conscious during the act but has no recall for the event later, much like a partial complex seizure.) Abstinence from alcohol is believed to extinguish future deviant behavior without specific focus on pedophilic urges (Forrest 1983). Families are treated with conjoint therapy and attendance at Al-Anon, pre-Alateen and Alateen (Whitfield 1980).

Sexual Adjustment in Male Homosexual Alcoholics

Denial of homosexuality was considered to be the principal cause of alcoholism at the turn of the century and for far too many years thereafter. Israelstam and Lambert (1983: 1086) refer to Karl Abraham's 1908 paper, first translated into English in 1926, as the first linkage. "Alcoholic drinks have an effect on the sexual instinct, for they dispel the resistances present and increase sexual activity. . . . To a healthy minded man any kind of tender contact with other men is repugnant. . . . These feelings are dispelled by alcohol" (Abraham 1926). Clark (1919) thought that alcoholic hallucinations were a form of persecution mania arising from unconscious and denied homosexuality.

Oral eroticism was considered a strong connection between alcoholism and homosexuality. Fellatio and alcoholism were both linked to longing for the mother's nipple (Israelstam and Lambert 1983: 1088-89).

Similar viewpoints prevailed and began to be refuted only in the 1950s. Levine (1953) had supported the latent homosexuality theory as an explanation for his finding of decreased sexual interest among 63 male and 16 female alcoholic patients.

Gerard (1955) thought that homosexuality and alcoholism had nothing to do with each other. He believed that alcohol and opiate addicts had been unable to develop a clear sex-role orientation, so that the fundamental problem was immaturity, not homosexuality. Levy (1940) stated that latent homosexual patterns could be found in any mixed group of psychiatric patients, and were not peculiar to groups of diagnosed alcoholics.

In the 1940s alcoholism was becoming a field of study in itself, led by Jellinek, who, with Browman, suggested that there were several types of alcoholism (Browman and Jellinek 1941). (Jellinek later developed an Institute of Alcohol Studies, now located at Rutgers.) The emphasis was on alcoholism as a disease as opposed to a personality defect. Branches of science other than psychoanalysis began to be applied.

Psychometric tests were utilized for the express purpose of objectifying data. The MMPI was given to members of AA by Hewitt (1943), who concluded that neither overt nor latent homosexuality was typical of the alcoholic. However, he noted that AA discouraged those whose appearance suggested homosexuality from becoming members! Several psychologists used masculine-feminine interest scales with alcoholic populations and controls, concluding that homosexuality is not an essential factor in alcoholism (Botwinick and Machover 1951; Machover et al. 1959). Botwinick and Machover pointed out that feminine interest is not necessarily a measure of homosexuality. Machover et al. (1959) studied remitted and unremitted populations and decided that homosexual trends were more common among recovered alcoholics, explaining that those who were no longer drinking were more secure and didn't have to disguise their homosexuality.

Sherfey (1955), a psychoanalyst, disagreed with the prevalent psychoanalytic view that homosexuality was the sole cause of alcoholism.

She studied male and female alcoholic populations of almost equal size (89 males and 73 females) and found 11 diagnostic groups, concluding that alcoholism is not a separate disease entity, and that it could be found as a symptom of several diseases.

The alcoholic male population treated at Silver Hill has been predominately heterosexual. Approximately 250 patients, half of whom are male, are admitted to the substance abuse service per year. Of those, there are usually from 10 to 15 male patients in the hospital occupying beds designated for substance abusers at any one time. (The remainder of the 22 beds are occupied by females.) Among the males, only 1 to 2 percent per population sample are homosexual. Half of these homosexual males are treated for addictions to drugs other than alcohol.

Most alcoholic males are heterosexual. Nevertheless the homosexual population of male alcoholics has special problems of adaptation that must be addressed in order to facilitate recovery from alcoholism. Fifield, DeCrescenzo, and Latham (1975) gathered self-report data from 200 patrons of gay bars in Los Angeles County, and interviewed 98 bartenders, 53 recovering gay alcoholics in rehabilitation centers, and 132 users of the Gay Community Services Center. He concluded that 31.4 percent of the Los Angeles homosexual and lesbian population were in need of treatment for alcoholism.

Nardi (1981) points out the diversity among gay alcoholics. "Some are 'in the closet' maintaining heterosexual identities while engaging in occasional homosexual behavior; some are 'out' and still adapting to their newly revealed identity; and others are openly and comfortably participating in a gay subculture." He focused on two types of gay alcoholics: those who were single and active in a gay community and those who were committed to another person and identified themselves as half of a couple. This summarizes the gay subculture in general.

Fenwick (1978) states that alcoholism among gay men is three times that of the general population because of gay bars, where single gay men are most likely to make contacts with prospective lovers as well as friends.

It has been my experience that, so long as the homosexuality is ego-syntonic, it can be discussed matter-of-factly in treating gay alcoholics. Trouble arises if a single homosexual is so preoccupied with finding a significant other that he doesn't focus on sobriety as his main priority in rehabilitation. This occurs also with patients whose relationships have recently terminated.

Small and Leach (1977), in their examination of 10 homosexual alcoholics, concluded that patients who "had come to terms with their homosexuality seemed to find it easier to accept the diagnosis of alcoholism and the need for abstinence" from alcohol "when the therapy did not demand that they become heterosexual." They suggest that gay alcoholics who insist that their fundamental problem is homosexuality are utilizing denial in deflecting attention away from their drinking. A similar point of view was expressed by Finnegan and Cook (1984). They add that homophobia in society adds to the difficulties that homosexuals face in accepting themselves and that therapists must be careful not to display this attitude. Display of self-help literature geared to adaptation of homosexual alcoholics in therapists' offices is suggested.

The adaptational problems facing sober homosexual alcoholics have to do largely with the social stigma of being homosexual superimposed on the stigma of being alcoholic. Patients need to find a support network in which they are free to speak about their homosexuality and their alcoholism. In large cities. Gay AA groups answer this need. With the advent of Gay AA chapters, homosexual men and women have a support system from which they had felt excluded in the early days of AA. In smaller towns or rural areas, it is difficult enough for a gay person to meet other gay people without also having to avoid social situations that revolve around drinking alcohol.

Gay couples face adjustment problems similar to those of heterosexual couples. The nonalcoholic member of the pair may feel conflicted about his partner's new abstinence from alcohol and need for avoidance of parties where alcohol is served. A partner who is angry and hurt about his lover's behavior when drinking may need to ventilate his feelings in couples therapy so that his anger will not sabatoge recovery. Erectile failure, ejaculatory incapacity, and diminished libido are problems for homosexual alcoholics as well as for heterosexuals. These dysfunctions diminish self-esteem, promote isolation, and compound the task of adjusting to a predominately heterosexual, nonalcoholic world.

Case Histories

Case 1. W., a 57-year-old man, entered the hospital for the second time because of daily drinking to the point of intoxication or passing out. Before passing out, he was almost invariably abusive verbally to his roommate. He was devastated when his lover of 20 years said that he wanted to end the relationship. Conjoint therapy was refused. His former lover said that he had given all he wanted to give to the relationship and it was over. W. could not picture a life without a sexual partner. He focused only on the problems a 57-year-old gay man would face in attracting another lover. All efforts at substance abuse rehabilitation were resisted, and W. seemed unwilling to see how his drinking had contributed to the breakup of the affair. Within two weeks he had become infatuated with a young, gay male patient and would talk only of his new relationship. He left the hospital in an elated state, with visions of the two supporting each other in AA. He quickly relapsed and has ignored advice to enter another rehabilitation center or to return to this one.

Case 2. E. said he always drank heavily but never noticed his drinking was problematic until his lover died. He required detoxification. He was being observed for clinical depression while in a drug-free state five days post-detox. Since his lover had died only a few months before, his grief reaction was acute. He could not concentrate on accepting the fact that he was addicted to alcohol and had no real interest in remaining alcohol-free. He felt old and unattractive and hated contemplating a single life. E. left the hospital against medical advice one week after having been admitted. He was allowed to leave because the doctor on call was satisfied that E. was not suicidal.

Case 3. M. was pressured into getting treatment by his lover. M. had lied to his friend, robbed him, and been verbally abusive while drunk. His lover was angry as well as concerned. M. rationalized at first by blaming his drinking on his roommate's absences which were due to occupational success and work demands. The treatment team and fellow patients changed his focus and forced him to confront his alcoholism. Conjoint therapy sessions with his lover, who was knowledgeable about substance abuse and very supportive of treatment efforts, helped to turn the attention back to substance abuse rehabilitation. The couple had had a sexual problem due to M.'s recent difficulty in maintaining an erection. This had led to increased performance insecurity which M. defended with anger. Abstinence from alcohol over a three-week period led to erection while masturbating and reassured M. that his impotence had been a consequence of alcohol, which, fortunately, was temporary. This reinforced fear of drinking. M. went to some Gay AA meetings in the neighborhood and was optimistic about having continued environmental support for remaining abstinent from alcohol.

Incidence of Sexual Deviance in Male Alcoholics

Very sparse data is available about the relationship of alcohol intoxication or chronic alcoholism to specific sexual deviations. In the absence of data, the usual controversy exists about whether the deviant behavior is the result of complex psychopathology (Nichols and Haines 1979; Mohr, Turner, and Terry 1964) or intoxication and/or alcoholism (Aarens et al. 1977). Mohr, Turner, and Terry, in a study of 247 pedophiles and exhibitionists, decided that alcohol does not play a significant role among youthful offenders, but exhibitionism in older men occurs in connection with chronic alcoholism and consequent organic deterioration. Nichols and Haines found that there is "dual denial" in the offender who suffers from sexual deviation and alcoholism. Mechanisms of dealing with the two diseases are similar and include rationalization and denial. Self-acknowledgement in support groups like AA and in treatment for populations of sexual offenders is thought to be useful.

Satyriasis was found in four men in a population of 1,200 alcoholics attending two rehabilitation centers. The sexual hyperactivity was considered to be an addiction (DeVito and Marozes 1981).

Recently the notion that compulsive sexual behavior is a separate addiction has become popular. Communities modeled after AA have been spreading across this country, Canada, and Europe with different names (Sexaholics Anonymous, Sexual Addicts Anonymous, and Sex and Love Addicts Anonymous; Carnes 1984). Some treatment centers have sprung up specifically to address compulsive sexual behavior. As with many compulsive behaviors such as bulimia, gambling, and abuse of drugs other than alcohol, the so-called sexual addiction often coexists with alcoholism. There are some distinctive characteristics that indicate whether or not a sexual behavior pattern qualifies as an addiction: secrecy and resulting excitement in leading a double life; exploitation of power as in pedophilia and incest, or sex with patients, subordinates, students; mood shifts having to do with shame and guilt; sex with people one does not know and/or does not like; the sense that one is violating ones own values (Carnes 1984: 12).

Case History

N., a 59-year-old dentist, was admitted because of cocaine and alcohol abuse. After a few days in the hospital, I began asking N. some routine questions pertaining to his sexual history. It seemed that N. had been suffering from sexual compulsions as well as substance abuse. He had barely escaped being arrested on two occasions. These incidents had involved fondling patients while they were under anesthesia. He was quite shaken about this. There were many other similar situations as well as innumerable extramarital affairs. Although he was deeply troubled by his own behavior he found himself unable to control it.

He talked nonstop; he had been on wild spending sprees, had temper outbursts, and was often contagiously humorous because of punning. All of these symptoms were still present after a two-week drug-free period and suggested the upswing of a bipolar disorder. He was placed on lithium carbonate and gradually his hypomanic symptoms lessened. He noted that his sexual urges had diminished and he could now control them.

It seemed that his aberrant sexual practices were linked to a mood disorder. Most of the time the solution is not so easily arrived at. If the deviance persists without the presence of alcohol, techniques such as aversive conditioning are useful. Such patients should be referred to specialized clinics for this treatment. Conditioning plus support from other patients with similar problems in group therapy is often a helpful combination. The alcoholism also has to be addressed. Total abstinence from alcohol and all other substances that are abused (i.e., sedative-hypnotics, opioids, amphetamines and cocaine, psychedelic drugs, and cannabis) should be advised. AA, in addition to group support from other sexual offenders, is recommended in order to reinforce the motivation to preserve a substance-free state.

Marital Sexual Adjustment in Male Alcoholics

Influence of Episodic Drinking as Opposed to Continuous Drinking on Adjustment

The quality of the marital relationship in families in which the husband is alcoholic depends on the impact that drinking behavior has on everyday functioning within the family. If the husband is emotionally inaccessible, negligent of personal hygiene, and/or relates to family members in a belligerent manner, it would seem obvious that this would have a negative effect on the marriage (Zweben 1986). Jacob, Dunn, and Leonard (1983) found a positive correlation between alcohol consumption and marital satisfaction among steady drinkers as compared with binge drinkers. Zweben suggests that sociobehavioral consequences may be worse among bingers than with steady drinkers. My own clinical experience would indicate that steady drinkers requiring hospitalization are often in deep interpersonal and occupational trouble. Perhaps Jacob's steady drinking sample had not yet reached that point. Jacob, Dunn, and Leonard (1983: 384) speculate that their finding might relate to unique sample characteristics in which the wives were highly adaptive. Steinglass (1981) studied 31 alcoholic families in their homes on nine separate occasions over six months. There were distinct interactional patterns observed during three family alcohol phases which Steinglass dubbed "stable wet, stable dry or transitional." Families in stable wet or transitional phases had rigid patterns of interaction, while those in the stable dry phase had flexible patterns.

Reciprocal Behavior in Spouse of Active Alcoholic

Experimental Evidence

Jacob, Dunn, and Leonard (1983) recruited eight alcoholic and eight nonalcoholic couples through newspaper advertisements. Alcoholism was established through history taking and the Michigan Alcoholism Screening Test. Couples were matched for age, family size, religion, years married, and occupation. Couples were in their forties, were non-Jewish, and had a mean of 5.4 nuclear family members, and the majority of husbands were administrators, salesmen, or skilled or semi-skilled workers. They filled out the Revealed Differences Questionnaire, which is a rank-ordered preference itemized test adapted from Bodin (Jacob, Dunn, and Leonard 1983: 469) and the Areas of Change Questionnaire (ACQ). The ACQ had been devised by Weiss (p. 470). The respondent asks a family member to modify a certain behavior and indicates to what degree it should be modified. These were administered in situations in which beverages were available and when they were not. Subjects were asked to fill out the sheets singly and then the RDQ was administered again for joint family discussion. Experimenters then presented the parents with two problem issues previously identified from the ACQ items and asked them to discuss and resolve the issues over a 15-minute period. There were two sessions of discussion, one of which took place under experimental drinking conditions. Half of the subjects received alcoholic beverages in each of the two sessions.

In the drinking session, the alcoholic husbands drank a mean of 1.56 oz. of absolute alcohol. The mean BAC post-session was 0.08 percent. Wives in the alcoholic group drank no alcohol in five cases. Three wives consumed a mean of 0.7 oz. Both spouses in the control group achieved BACs of only 0.01-0.04.

In the family interactions, alcoholic fathers exhibited less leadership and assertiveness in problem-solving than nonalcoholic fathers. Mothers in the alcoholic families were more directive than mothers in the control group. In alcoholic families, spouse interactions "reflected greater negativity in the drink vs. no-drink condition" (p. 480). The authors recommend that further studies should attend to key variables such as amount of alcohol consumed and the relative importance of psychosocial as opposed to pharmacological effects of alcohol (Jacob et al. 1981). Billings et al. (1979) reported little difference between alcoholic couples and nonalcoholic distressed couples as compared with controls. Both groups of distressed couples displayed fewer problem-solving responses and "engaged in more negative and hostile acts." In contrast with Jacob's findings and previous reports (Steinglass et al. 1977; Steinglass 1981; Burton and Kaplan 1968), interaction in the alcoholic group didn't change in drinking versus non-drinking situations.

Frankenstein, Hay, and Nathan (1985) studied the effects of intoxication in eight alcoholic couples who were motivated for treatment. Two of the eight alcoholic spouses were female and six were male. The mean age was 41 and alcohol had been a problem for an average of 11.1 years. They were all well educated. Four had graduated from college and two had advanced degrees. All had completed high school. Couples received either alcohol or no alcohol in two sessions a week apart. They were seated in a mock living room "close enough to achieve physical contact." They discussed the alcohol problem, a major marital problem, and a minor marital problem. Couples were randomly assigned to predetermined topic sequences. In half of the sessions, the alcoholics reached blood levels of 10 mg/dl. In contrast to the studies previously cited in this chapter, couples expressed themselves verbally in a more positive manner when the alcoholic spouse was drinking. The nonalcoholic spouses doubled their rate of positive verbal behavior in the drinking sessions. "Alcoholics spoke more and tended to make more problem-solving statements while intoxicated than while sober." In terms of nonverbal behavior, alcoholic spouses were more negative than their partners. The authors suggest that alcohol may produce benefits in alcoholic couples' style of interaction which reinforce drinking. However, the authors point out that variables such as gender of the alcoholic, the level of marital satisfaction or the alcoholic's tolerance level must be considered. The BAL achieved was relatively low and "high tolerance for alcohol may have produced an effect on interactions quite apart from social-learning or systems theory implications." The clinical implications of the results are that the benefits to the relationship derived from drinking must be restored in treatment under sober conditions.

Beliefs of Substance-Abuse Clinicians and Self-Help Group Members in AA and Al-Anon

The views can be summarized as follows: The defense mechanisms utilized by many alcoholics in reference to their disease are rationalization and denial. Alcoholics with terminal liver disease, revoked driving licenses, lost relationships, and lost jobs can still insist that the diagnosis is something other than alcoholism ("I'm in the hospital because of the stress I've been under lately.").

Bargaining goes on as it does when people are faced with any life-threatening illness ("I can't be an alcoholic if I only drink wine, never drink in the morning, am still a valued employee, etc.").

As Al-Anon teaches, spouses adapt with the same defense mechanisms. They find other reasons for the husband's behavior and often refuse to admit that there is a problem and thus manifest denial. Until she is almost totally burned out, the wife of an alcoholic unintentionally facilitates drinking by building up a conspiracy of silence. The problem is not discussed with the children, friends, or other family members. If her husband gets drunk she covers up for him as best she can. Frequently this results in tremendous feelings of neglect, fears of abandonment, and resentment. Most untutored spouses of alcoholics believe that their partners cannot drink this way and still love them.

Often the wife of an alcoholic is convinced that the drinking is her fault and that it is therefore her responsibility to prevent recurrences of drinking. This unrealistic guilt leads to an anxious vigilance which produces resentment from the husband because of "nagging."

The wife also feels that she must protect her children from her husband's emotional neglect and verbal or physical abuse. Apart from the children, wives of alcoholics are frequently the victims of physical abuse inflicted by their intoxicated husbands. It would follow that the reactions produced by the husband's drinking behavior are not conducive to promoting sexual desire in wives. Alcoholic husbands may then retaliate by seeking sexual satisfaction in protracted affairs or one-night stands.

In *Getting Them Sober*, a practical guide for spouses of alcoholics, Toby Rice Drews devotes an appendix to sex and alcohol (Drews 1980). She describes what she believes to be repetitive and typical behaviors in the sexual lives of women married to alcoholics. Sex and alcohol have become "almost a contradiction in terms." If the husband isn't passed out, he is trying to prove he's potent, even while exhausted. "Or he is so selfish, he always wants you to perform oral sex. Or when he does sometimes focus on you, it's so mechanical that you get depressed." If the wife then tries to talk with her husband about her feelings, he withdraws, stalking out indignantly, or promising to do better and then leaving. The silent treatment is the worst barrier to discussion. Drews points out that sex is the last part of the relationship to break down because if that goes the wife feels that her entire marriage is threatened. Husbands not only throw up, pass out, or become impotent but they also threaten success with other women. Drews advises that wives realize that they don't deserve to feel guilty about the relationship. She counsels wives to refuse sex when they don't want it and assert their own needs when they are feeling sexual, regardless of their husband's complaints and self-absorption. She recommends also that wives stop hoping that their husbands will learn and change, since active alcoholics do not learn.

Philosophy of Al-Anon: Detachment with Love

Al-Anon teaches relatives of alcoholics to relinquish responsibility for maintaining abstinence from alcohol. AA has a 12-step program of recovery with principles to which successful AA members refer the rest of their lives. Al-Anon's steps are identical. The first step in AA is that the alcoholic has no power over alcohol. This does not imply that one can't help it if one drinks. It means that drinking makes the alcoholic's life unmanageable and that the amount of alcohol consumed cannot be controlled; therefore the alcoholic should remain abstinent from alcohol. In Al-Anon, members are taught that they are powerless to affect the spouse's drinking. They cannot control it and should not feel guilty, try to prevent it, or cover it up. Responsibility for drinking or not drinking is entirely in the hands of the alcoholic. Wives need not withdraw affection but should develop self-realization by gaining satisfaction in other areas of their lives.

Influence on Marital Sexual Adjustment of Abstinence in Recovering Male Alcoholics

The Hazelden Foundation counsels that the main obstacle to recovery of sexual intimacy is the gender type-casting from which our society is slowly emerging. Male stereotypes such as James Bond promote expectations of being sexually aggressive and attractive to many women. Alcohol is thought to provide a way of living up to this image by making sexual overtures possible. During recovery the male is beset with memories of sexual dysfunction while intoxicated, which reinforces sexual performance fears. Men are advised to examine sex-role stereotypes along with their spouses and develop a more equal relationship based on sharing and intimacy (McFarland 1984). Similar advice is offered by Weinberg (1977) and Ackerman (1986). Davis, Purcell, and Burnham (1979) administered sex-role inventory tests as well as the MMPI to 69 males who were 7 to 10 days post-detoxification from alcohol and nonpsychotic. The sex-role inventory was a measure of androgyny versus non-androgyny. High scorers on the androgyny scale had scores on the MMPI reflecting a hopeful, positive self-concept, whereas "non-androgynous subjects" scored higher on subtests of the MMPI, reflecting psychological distress. This implies that men who perceived themselves as fulfilling a masculine role had higher self-esteem compared with those who did not.

Moos and Moos (1984) studied 54 families of recovered alcoholics and compared them with 51 families in which the husband had relapsed and with matched controls. Families in which relapse had occurred showed less cohesion, expressiveness, and recreational orientation than recovering families and matched controls. Quality of marital sexual adjustment per se was not discussed. Interestingly, Frank, Anderson, and Rubenstein (1978) examined the frequency of sexual dysfunction among a population of self-described "happily married" couples and found 40 percent of males with erectile and ejaculatory dysfunction and 50 percent with lack of interest in sex. This was not a result of age since the men were in their mid-thirties. In 5 to 10 percent of cases one partner was not aware of dysfunction in the other. Premature ejaculation was more frequently a problem than ejaculatory delay or failure. The latter is more often associated with alcoholism, but drinking histories were not mentioned.

Kaufman and Pattison (1981) reviewed some typical interactional patterns within families of male alcoholics and suggested the adaptation of family therapy techniques specific for each type of constellation. They observed that the spouse may no longer fight with her husband about his drinking but "about whether he will resume drinking." In families that are relatively intact and loving despite the father's drinking, the focus should be on treating the alcoholism rather than on changing defensive structure. In some families, maintaining a "wet" system, wherein the drinking continues, serves as a mechanism for discharging tension. Such families are engaged in dwelling on the past rather than on problem-solving. Getting family members disengaged from enmeshment via Al-Anon, AA, and Alateen is advised. Disintegrated families in which there has been job loss and separation can be reintegrated once sobriety has been established. In these situations the past is reviewed in order to make future plans. An attempt is made to reestablish mutual respect even if separation continues. In terminal stages of family deterioration, the alcoholic has been isolated from his family for many years. In such cases, the alcoholic is encouraged to form a new extended family through AA, church, and recreational and avocational clubs.

Case History

Case 1. Bill J., aged 59, entered the hospital because of chronic alcoholism. He and his wife had been fighting verbally for years about his drinking. He was persuaded to take early retirement from his firm because of frequent absenteeism.

He and his wife had not had sexual intercourse for years, even though he was not impotent. Their interactions were nearly always combative verbally. Bill had never struck his wife. As a matter of fact, Mrs. J. always played the aggressor. Their college-aged son and daughter were polarized; the son sided with his father and the daughter with her mother.

Bill's wife attended a series of four didactic multiple-family groups in which an attempt was made to educate her about alcoholism and utilization of Al-Anon. She and Bill also met with his psychiatrist and his counselor in two individual sessions. The children were out of state and unable to attend. In both individual sessions, Ruth J. acted as a prosecuting attorney. She continued to dwell on her husband's morose, withdrawn drinking behavior and was entirely distrustful of his efforts to stop drinking. While we acknowledged that she had suffered, an attempt was made to point out her aggressive style and to encourage Bill to be assertive in his own behalf. Ruth did become active in Al-Anon and joined while Bill was in the hospital. Bill discovered that he derived relief from confiding in his sponsor and attending AA.

Neither Bill nor Ruth have chosen to leave each other in spite of repeated mutual threats to separate.

Case 2. Mark T., a 45-year-old, highly successful business executive, sought help after learning about his disorderly behavior while in an alcoholic blackout during an out-of-town and very crucial annual business meeting. He elected to seek help himself but was also forcibly urged to by his firm.

He and his wife had always enjoyed a close relationship. Sexually, they were compatible and active. Except for recent sleepiness on weekends as a result of all-weekend drinking, Jane T. had not experienced any unpleasant consequences of Mark's alcohol abuse. It was during out-of-town trips that Mark's behavior had become problematic for his company.

Although he had improved the profits of his division dramatically, he was fired with a separation contract.

When his wife, Jane, became involved in conjoint treatment sessions, the first interviews were centered around her anger at the way the company had treated her husband. She did not want Mark to tell their children because she feared it would jeopardize their relationship.

She attended daily films and discussions about alcohol along with Mark and began to understand her husband's alcoholism. She was urged to join Al-Anon and went to a meeting on the Silver Hill premises.

Mark and Jane had yet to decide whether or not they would inform the children. Mark's mother only recently informed him about his paternal grandfather's alcoholism. He believed that telling the children was better than operating in secret. He hoped it would also cause them to limit their drinking, thus preventing future cases of familial alcoholism.

The most distressing problem was reemployment. Jane feared that inactivity would lead to more drinking. Mark would have good severence pay and business acumen to prepare him for the future. He left the hospital with a strong attachment to AA, a schedule of meetings in his home area, and a number of ideas for new business ventures. On the face of it, Jane did not blame Mark for his alcoholism and the relationship remained cohesive.

Treatment Goal of "Controlled Drinking"— Is Marital Adjustment Better?

In the 1970s, after the initial Rand report on treatment outcome for alcoholics, it was suggested that some alcoholics could be treated with a goal of modified drinking as opposed to total abstinence (Armor, Polich, and Stambul 1978; Polich, Armor, and Braiker 1980). Since small amounts of alcohol are viewed by many social drinkers and alcoholics as social lubricants, it had been hypothesized that marital adjustment post-treatment would be easier for those who continued to drink moderately. Follow-up studies of alcoholics in the early stages of recovery supported this by default, since, in the initial dry stage, alcoholics had a tendency to be depressed with a poor level of adjustment. Longer-term recovered alcoholics, with a minimum of four years of sobriety, were more socially inhibited than controls but had self-acceptance, a sense of well-being, and social maturity mid-way between controls and early-stage recoverers (Kurtines, Ball, and Wood 1978).

Finney and Moos (1981) studied populations of abstinent alcoholics, moderate drinkers immediately post-treatment, and moderate drinkers who began to drink after a period of abstinence lasting six months or more. Early moderate drinkers returned to families who were more involved in joint recreational activities, but their work environments were lower in peer cohesion and staff support than the work environments of abstainers. Only one of the early moderate drinkers was continuing to drink moderately at the 18-month follow-up. The other six had relapsed and were drinking heavily. There was a relapse rate of 56 percent in the late moderate drinkers. The spouses of the moderate drinkers were more likely to drink heavily than the spouses of abstainers. This suggests that both work environments and immediate social environments of moderate drinkers promoted relapse. Moderate drinkers were thought to have been overconfident and less aware of the severity of alcoholism than abstainers. The authors conclude nevertheless that there should be some treatment programs that utilize moderate drinking as a goal, because such programs would attract alcoholics who cannot abstain.

Early-stage recovery is a difficult process, since it requires intense concentration on the task of remaining abstinent from alcohol. At this point spouses may become resentful, understandably, about playing second fiddle once more, this time to abstinence instead of the bottle. However, there are long-term rewards in living with a sober alcoholic if the wife is willing to wait it out, while getting support in Al-Anon with or without additional therapy. Moos, Finney, and Gamble (1982) studied 429 families treated at five residential facilities. They concluded that wives of recovered alcoholics had suffered effects of stress which diminished when the spouse was successfully treated. There was "no support" for the hypothesis that wives of recovered alcoholics were more disturbed than wives of nonalcoholics. There was lack of support also for the notion that their functioning was detrimentally affected by their spouses' efforts at recovery.

Several looks at post-treatment populations verify that the percentage of alcoholics who can maintain controlled drinking is small (Helzer et al. 1985; Edwards et al. 1983). It would seem that the advantages of marital adjustment with a treatment goal of controlled drinking are short-term, except in rare cases. In addition, mortality and morbidity rates for abstinent alcoholics are significantly less than for those who continue to drink (Helzer et al. 1985; Edwards et al. 1983; Barr et al. 1984).

Sexual Adjustment in Recovering, Single, Male Alcoholics

Admonitions of Therapists and AA

Single alcoholics are advised to look for partners in supermarkets rather than in bars (Weinberg 1977). Fear of rejection is considered a great obstacle to starting conversations without the aid of alcohol. Training in self-assertiveness is advised. In AA, new members are instructed not to begin serious relationships for the first six months to a year after joining. Williams (1976) suggests a moratorium on new close personal relationships in the early stages of recovery. Rejection, anxiety about sexual performance without alcohol, and shifting the focus from abstinence to developing the relationship are cited by substance-abuse counselors as frequent triggers for relapse in newly recovered alcoholics.

"Romance on the campus" is a frequent problem in residential substance abuse rehabilitation programs. Rarely do such romances lead to continued mutual support and recovery for both partners. Usually, neither member of the romantic team is able to stay sober because both have become preoccupied with infatuation for each other and have lost sight of the reason for hospitalization, which is to learn how to remain abstinent from alcohol.

Sexual dysfunctions compound the difficulties faced by single males. Longing for successful relationships while constantly remembering sexual performance failures can lead to alcohol as an anesthetic for anxiety, even though alcohol will probably impair performance still further.

Case history 1. Joe W., aged 38, had been abstinent from alcohol and active in AA for a year after a 28-day rehabilitation program. He then decided he should date again and became attracted to his future wife, whom he took out to dinner. He found himself unable to admit to her that he had a drinking problem and had his first glass of wine on their first date. After they had been married for three months following a whirlwind courtship, Joe developed gastrointestinal bleeding as a result of gastric irritation induced by alcohol. He was a highly valued member of his engineering firm, and his partners urged him to return for treatment after lateness, absenteeism, and incomplete projects began to characterize his work performance.

Although being around alcohol triggered in Joe an immense craving for a drink, his wife saw any curtailment of their social life as a great imposition. Shortly after Joe was discharged from the hospital, he and his wife were separated.

Case history 2. Ted, aged 30, had relapsed for two years after six months of sobriety. He had been suffering from erectile failure during attempts at intercourse since the age of 18. Consumption of two six-packs of beer a day had also begun at age 18. When not drinking, Ted was able to masturbate with full erection and complete ejaculation. It had never occurred to him that he had not been drinking while masturbating and had always been drinking when with women. He developed severe performance anxiety, which hampered his ability to have intercourse during his first six-month recovery period.

During the second rehabilitation attempt, Ted's general lack of assertiveness in speaking up at AA meetings and in groups about neutral, nonsexual subjects became manifest. He became convinced that he needed to practice stating his needs and asking for help in order to enhance his self-esteem. He obtained an AA sponsor, who accompanied him to his apartment and helped him throw out his remaining cases of beer. He knew he would never have been able to resist his well-stocked refrigerator if he had faced the beer without a buddy who understood his problem.

Because of erectile incompetence, his sexual desire had decreased while drinking. He noted increased masturbation while in the hospital but decided he would concentrate on becoming sober for the next 6- to 12-month period, since attempts at intercourse might tempt him to drink if he were not able to perform. It was agreed that he would see a psychiatrist specializing in sexual therapy after six months of sobriety, and he was given a list of several whom he could consult. He seemed relieved that he could put off addressing his sexual problem for a while: "I'm under less pressure knowing that I don't have to perform. I just have to stay sober."

Recently, two self-help groups dealing with male impotence have formed: Impotents Anonymous, for those who are impotent, and I-Anon, for their partners (*Psychiatric News*, January 3, 1986, p. 6).

Adjustment in Homosexual Alcoholics Who Are Abstinent from Alcohol

Finnegan and Cook (1984) state a truth of which many therapists treating homosexuals are well aware. Not only do homosexuals have to face a homophobic society but also they must contend with internalized homophobia. They have most often been brought up by homophobic parents and lived among homophobic peers, thus absorbing society's views of homosexuality as their very own. There is added defensiveness in rehabilitating homosexuals who are suspicious that others are talking about their sexual orientation. Alcohol enhances their ability to isolate and anesthetize pain. Furthermore, alcohol serves as a means to socialize with other homosexuals.

As previously mentioned in this chapter ("Sexual Adjustment in Male Homosexual Alcoholics"), homosexuals can be successfully rehabilitated. However, it is much more difficult for single homosexual alcoholics who are preoccupied with finding an antedote to loneliness. As with male heterosexuals, concentration within Gay AA support groups on staying sober has to be the number one priority for quite some time. If it is not, and infatuation or obsession with obtaining a mate supervenes, relapse is extremely likely to occur (see case histories under "Sexual Adjustment," above).

Homosexuals who are conflicted about their sexual orientation need psychotherapy with a non-homophobic therapist who is also knowledgeable about substance abuse. These patients must continue to remain sober if they are ever to resolve their sexual conflicts since, as is said in AA, "There is nothing that alcohol doesn't make worse." If a patient does not wish to identify himself with homosexuals, he may be more comfortable at regular AA meetings, which have become less homophobic in recent years.

EXPERIMENTAL INVESTIGATIONS

Effect of Blood Alcohol Level on Penile Tumescence

Wilson, Lawson, and Abrams (1978) studied the effect of alcohol in varying dosages on eight male alcoholics chosen from respondents to a newspaper advertisement. They were examined and interviewed to determine that they met criteria for the experiment (i.e., fulfilled a diagnosis of alcoholism, had no neurologic or physical impairment, had no coexisting psychiatric illness, and were not taking drugs other than alcohol). None had a history of sexual dysfunction. They each received four doses of alcohol in counterbalanced order, prior to viewing non-erotic and erotic films. Measures of penile tumescence obtained with a penile plethysmograph showed a significant decrease in tumescence with increasing alcohol doses during the heterosexual and homosexual films; the effect was linear.

Effect of Expectation on Penile Tumescence with Varying Blood Levels

Expectations about the effect of alcohol on sexual arousal and behavior "were discrepant with these physiological findings" (Wilson, Lawson, and Abrams 1978: 609). Subjects believed that alcohol would have no effect on their sexual arousal or would enhance arousal. At BALs beyond 40 to 50 mg percent, there is a negative effect of alcohol on tumescence, regardless of expectation. This becomes especially manifest at levels of 100 mg percent. The homosexual films were shown to determine whether or not there were differential effects of alcohol on conventional heterosexual as opposed to "deviant" (p. 614) sexual stimuli. Subjects showed less arousal in response to the homosexual films than to the heterosexual films at all four BALs. The design was balanced placebo in nature, so that expectancy was controlled.

Interestingly, Wincze and Qualls (1984) examined sexual arousal in eight nonalcoholic male and eight nonalcoholic female homosexuals and demonstrated greatest physiological and subjective response to sexually explicit same-gender homosexual films. These data would suggest that films portraying sexual activity that is deviant to the viewers are not as stimulating as are films depicting activity congruent with the viewers' sexual orientation.

SUMMARY

Endocrinological and physiological data document clearly the negative impact of chronic alcoholism on sexual functioning in males.

Psychosocial effects remain controversial. Earlier literature is based on the assumption that an underlying sexual orientation conflict is the etiology of alcoholism. This view is still held by some authors, who then conclude that the social disruption in their study populations is a consequence of ego-dystonic homosexual preference rather than of alcoholism itself. Many, including this writer, do not agree. There is ample evidence cited in this chapter that would indicate that sexual dysfunction in alcoholics is produced by the toxic hormonal and neurological action of the drug alcohol. There is no need to invoke pre-morbid sexual conflict to explain it.

The chicken-or-egg controversy prevails in the literature in reference to sex crimes and sexual deviance. Some data indicate that there is a high correlation between rape and incest, and other data contradict this. Modern studies suggest that, although drinking is associated with rape in many cases, few alcoholics are rapists. Opinions are less united in regard to the correlation between alcoholism and incest. There is very little data in general about pedophilia. Sexual deviance does not seem to be prevalent among alcoholics, with the exception of compulsive sexual intercourse in the form of an "addiction" (see "Marital Sexual Adjustment in Male Alcoholics," this chapter).

Sexual adjustment in male homosexuals is complicated by the combined social stigma of being homosexual and alcoholic. Rehabilitation programs must accept the homosexual's sexual orientation matter-of-factly and address the alcoholism. Support groups in the community, particularly Gay AA chapters, can be enlisted in the recovery process. Single homosexuals have a much more difficult adjustment than do alcoholic partners of an intact couple. This is often true for heterosexuals as well.

The impact of alcoholism on marriages has been hotly debated. Some workers suggest that alcohol provides a focus for marital interaction, which treatment threatens. Other data suggest clear dysfunctional family and marital interaction during "wet" as opposed to "dry" phases of alcoholism. Obviously there are different types of interactional systems in alcoholic marriages just as there are in nonalcoholic ones. In early stages of the disease of alcoholism, families are often stable and affectionate, unless they are dysfunctional because of coexisting problems. In later stages, there is marked disruption. Treatment approaches need to be adapted to suit particular sets of family circumstances.

Finally, AA, Al-Anon, and Alateen have folk wisdom that applies accurately to many situations faced by alcoholics and their families.

In this chapter, I have attempted to demonstrate that some of the advice given by members of these organizations can be substantiated by data from clinical studies.

REFERENCES

Aarens, M., T. Cameron, J. Roizen, R. Roizen, R. Room, D. Schneberk, and D. Wingard. 1977. "Alcohol, Casualties and Crime." Report no. C-18, *Selected Studies on the Societal-Epidemiological Aspects of Alcohol Use and Alcohol-Related Problems* (Berkeley, CA: National Institute on Alcohol Abuse and Alcoholism, November).

Abel, E. 1985. *Psychoactive Drugs and Sex* (New York: Plenum Press).

Abraham, K. 1926. "The Psychological Relationship Between Sexuality and Alcoholism." *Internat. J. Psychoanal.* 7:1-10.

Ackerman, H. 1986. "Real Alcoholics Can Eat Quiche—Strategies for Working with Men's Gender Issues in Treatment." *Focus on Family* (May-June):24-25.

Amir, M. 1967. "Alcohol and Forcible Rape." *Br. J. Addict.* 62:219-32.

Armor, D. J., J. M. Polich, and H. Stambul. 1978. *Alcoholism and Treatment* (New York: Wiley).

Awad, G. A. 1976. "Father-Son Incest: A Case Report." *J. Nerv. Ment. Dis.* 162:135-39.

Barr, H. L., D. Antes, D. J. Ottenberg, and A. Rosen. 1984. "Mortality of Treated Alcoholics and Drug Addicts: The Benefits of Abstinence." *J. Stud. Alcohol* 45:440-52.

Bhalla, V., C. Chen, and M. Granaprakasam. 1979. "Effects of *In Vivo* Administration of Human Chorionic Gonadotropin and Ethanol on the Processes of Testicular Receptor Depletion and Replacement." *Life Sci.* 24:1315-24.

Billings, A. G., M. Kessler, C. Gomberg, and S. Weiner. 1979. "Marital Conflict Resolution of Alcoholic and Nonalcoholic Couples During Drinking and Nondrinking Sessions." *J. Stud. Alcohol* 40, no. 3: 183-85.

Botwinick, J., and S. Machover. 1951. "A Psychometric Examination of Latent Homosexuality in Alcoholism." *Q. J. Stud. Alcohol* 12: 268-72.

Browman, K. M., and E. M. Jellinek. 1941. "Alcoholic Mental Disorders." *Q. J. Stud. Alcohol* 2:312-90.

Burton, G., and H. Kaplan. 1968. "Sexual Adjustment and Behavior of Married Alcoholics." *Q. J. Stud. Alcohol* 29:603-9.

Cadoret, R. J., E. Troughton, and T. W. O'Gorman. 1987. "Genetics and Environmental Factors in Alcohol Abuse and Antisocial Personality." *J. Stud. Alcohol* 48, no. 1:1-8.

Carnes, P. J. 1984. "Sexual Addictions." *Focus on the Family* and *Chemical Dependency* (July-August):10-12.

Cavallin, H. 1966. "Incestuous Fathers: A Clinical Report." *Am. J. Psychiatr.* 122:1132-38.

Chiao, Y., D. Johnston, J. Gavaler, and D. Van Thiel. 1981. "Effect of Chronic Ethanol Feeding on Testicular Content of Enzymes Required for Testosteronogenesis." *Alcoholism: Clin. Exptl. Res.* 5: 230-36.

Chiao, Y., and D. Van Thiel. 1983. "Biochemical Mechanisms that Contribute to Alcohol-Induced Hypogonadism in the Male." *Alcoholism: Clin. Exptl. Res.* 7:131-34.

Cicero, T. J. 1980. "Common Mechanisms Underlying the Effects of Ethanol and the Narcotics on Neuroendocrine Function." In *Advances in Substance Abuse*, vol. 1, edited by N. K. Mello (Greenwich, CT: JAI Press), pp. 201-54.

Cicero, T. J., and R. Bell. 1980. "Effects of Ethanol and Acetaldehyde on the Biosynthesis of Testosterone in the Rodent Testes." *Biochem. Biophys. Res. Commun.* 94:814-19.

Cicero, T. J., R. Bell, E. Meyer, and T. Badger. 1980. "Ethanol and Acetaldehyde Directly Inhibit Testicular Steriodogenesis." *J. Pharmacol. Exptl. Ther.* 213:228-33.

Clark, L. R. 1919. "Some Psychological Aspects of Alcoholism." *N.Y. Med. J.* 109:930-33.

Cloninger, C. R., M. Bohman, and S. Sigvardsson. 1981. "Inheritance of Alcohol Abuse: A Cross-Fostering Analysis of Adopted Men." *Arch. Gen. Psychiatr.* 38, no. 8:861-68.

Davis, W. E., S. A. Purcell, and R. A. Burnham. 1979. "Alcoholism, Sex-Role Orientation and Psychological Distress." *J. Clin. Psychol.* 35: 209-12.

DeVito, R. A., and R. J. Marozes. 1981. "The Alcoholic Satyr." *Sexuality Disability* 4:234-45.

Douglas, J. J., and C. P. Nutter. 1986. "Treatment-Related Change in Sex Roles of Addicted Men and Women." *J. Stud. Alcohol* 47, no. 3:201-5.

Drews, T. R. 1980. *Getting Them Sober: A Guide for Those Who Live with an Alcoholic*, vol. 1 (South Plainfield, NJ: Bridge Publishing), pp. 193-99.

Eagon, P., L. Porter, J. Gavaler, K. Egler, and D. Van Thiel. 1981. "Effect of a Male-Specific Hepatic Estrogen Binding Protein: A Possible Mechanism for Feminization." *Alcoholism: Clin. Exptl. Res.* 5: 183-87.

Edwards, G., A. Duckett, E. Oppenheimer, M. Sheehan, and C. Taylor. 1983. "What Happens to Alcoholics?" *Lancet* July 30, pp. 268-71.

Ellingboe, J., and C. Varinelli. 1979. "Ethanol Inhibits Testosterone Biosynthesis by Direct Action on Leydig Cells." *Res. Comm. Chem. Pathol. Pharmacol.* 24:87-102.

Fenwick, R. D. 1978. "Alcohol and Other Drugs." In *The Advocate Guide to Gay Health*, edited by R. D. Fenwick (New York: E.P. Dutton).

Fifield, L. 1980. "Alcoholism and the Gay Community." Paper presented at the National Council on Alcoholism Annual Meeting, Seattle.

Fifield, L., T. A. DeCrescenzo, and J. Latham. 1975. "Alcoholism and the Gay Community." Summary of "On My Way to Nowhere: Alienated, Isolated, Drunk: An Analysis of Gay Acohol Abuse and an Evaluation of Alcoholism Rehabilitation Services for the Los Angeles County" (Los Angeles, CA: Gay Community Services Center).

Filmore, K. M. 1985. "Social Victims of Drinking." *Br. J. Addict.* 80: 307-14.

Finkelhor, D. 1980. "Sex Among Siblings: A Survey on Prevalence, Variety, and Effects." *Arch. Sex. Behav.* 9, no. 3:171-94.

Finnegan, D. G., and D. Cook. 1984. "Special Issues Affecting the Treatment of Male Homosexual and Lesbian Alcoholics." In *Alcoholism and Sexual Dysfunction: Issues in Clinical Management*, edited by D. J. Powell (New York: The Haworth Press), pp. 85-99.

Finney, J. W., and R. H. Moos. 1981. "Characteristics and Prognosis of Alcoholics Who Become Moderate Drinkers and Abstainers After Treatment." *J. Stud. Alcohol* 42:94-105.

Forrest, G. 1983. *Alcoholism and Human Sexuality* (Springfield, IL: Charles C Thomas).

Frank, E., C. Anderson, and P. Rubenstein. 1978. "Frequency of Sexual Dysfunction in 'Normal' Couples." *N. Engl. J. Med.* 299, no. 3: 111-15.

Frankenstein, W., W. Hay, and P. Nathan. 1985. "Effect of Intoxication on Alcoholics' Marital Problem Solving." *J. Stud. Alcohol* 46, no. 1:1-5.

Gagnon, J. H. 1977. *Human Sexualities* (Oakland, NJ: Scott, Foresman), pp. 310-11.

Gallant, D. M. 1986. "A Study of the Victims of Alcohol Abusers." *Alcoholism: Clin. Exptl. Res.* 10, no. 3:358-59.

Gerard, D. I. 1955. "Intoxication and Addiction: Psychiatric Observations on Alcoholism and Opiate Drug Addiction." *Q. J. Stud. Alcohol* 16:681-89.

Goodwin, D. 1985. "Alcoholism and Genetics . . . The Sins of the Fathers." *Arch. Gen. Psychiatr.* 42:171-74.

Gordon, G. G., A. Southren, and C. Lieber. 1978. "The Effects of Alcoholic Liver Disease and Alcohol Ingestion on Sex Hormone Levels." *Alcoholism: Clin. Exptl. Res.* 2:259-63.

Gordon, G. G., A. Southren, and C. Lieber. 1979. "Hypogonadism and Feminization in the Male: A Triple Effect of Alcohol." *Alcoholism: Clin. Exptl. Res.* 3:210-12.

Gordon, G. G., J. Olivo, F. Rafii, and A. Southren. 1975. "Conversion of Androgens to Estrogens in Cirrhosis of the Liver." *J. Clin. Endocrinol. Metab.* 40:1018-26.

Gordon, G. G., A. Southren, J. Vittek, and C. Lieber. 1979a. "The Effect of Alcohol Ingestion on Hepatic Aromatase Activity and Plasma Steroid Hormones in the Rat." *Metabolism* 28:20-24.

Gordon, G. G., J. Vittek, R. Ho, W. Rosenthal, A. Southren, and C. Lieber. 1979b. "Effect of Chronic Alcohol Use on Hepatic Testosterone Alpha A-Ring Reductase in the Baboon and in the Human Being." *Gastroenterology* 77:110-14.

Gordon, G. G., J. Vittek, A. Southren, P. Munnang, and C. Lieber. 1980. "Effect of Chronic Alcohol Ingestion on the Biosynthesis of Steroids in Rat Testicular Homogenates *in vitro*." *Endocrinology* 106: 1880-85.

Helzer, J., L. N. Robins, J. R. Taylor, K. Carey, R. Miller, T. Coombs-Orme, and A. Farmer. 1985. "The Extent of Long-Term Moderate Drinking Among Alcoholics Discharged from Medical and Psychiatric Treatment Facilities." *N. Engl. J. Med.* June 27, pp. 1678-82.

Hewitt, C. C. 1943. "A Personality Study of Alcohol Addiction." *Q. J. Stud. Alcohol* 4:368-86.

Israelstam, S., and S. Lambert. 1983. "Homosexuality as a Cause of Alcoholism: A Historical Review." *Internat. J. Addict.* 18, no. 8:1085-1108.

Jacob, T., N. J. Dunn, and K. Leonard. 1983. "Patterns of Alcohol Abuse and Family Stability." *Alcoholism: Clin. Exptl. Res.* 7, no. 4:382-85.

Jacob, T., D. Ritchey, J. Cvitkovic, and H. Blau. 1981. "Communication Styles of Alcoholic and Nonalcoholic Families When Drinking and Not Drinking." *J. Stud. Alcohol* 42, no. 5:466-82.

Jensen, S. B. 1979. "Sexual Customs and Dysfunction in Alcoholics: Part II." *Br. J. Sex. Med.* 6:30-34.

Johnston, D. E., Y. B. Chiao, J. S. Gavaler, and D. Van Thiel. 1981. "Inhibition of Testosterone Synthesis by Ethanol and Acetaldehyde." *Biochem. Pharmacol.* 30:1827-31.

Kaufman, E., and E. M. Pattison. 1981. "Differential Methods of Family Therapy in the Treatment of Alcoholism." *J. Stud. Alcohol* 42, no. 11:951-71.

Kolodny, R. C., W. H. Masters, and V. E. Johnson. 1979. *Textbook of Sexual Medicine* (Boston, MA: Little, Brown).

Kreuz, L. E., and R. M. Rose. 1972. "Assessment of Aggressive Behavior and Plasma Testosterone in a Young Criminal Population." *Psychosomat. Med.* 24:321.

Kurtines, W. M., L. R. Ball, and G. H. Wood. 1978. "Personality Characteristics of Long-Term Recovered Alcoholics: A Comparative Analysis." *J. Consulting Criminal Psychol.* 46, no. 5:971-77.

Lemere, F., and J. W. Smith. 1973. "Alcohol-Induced Sexual Impotence." *Am. J. Psychol.* 130, no. 2:212-13.

Lester, R., P. K. Eagon, and D. Van Thiel. 1979. "Feminization of the Alcoholic: The Estrogen/Testosterone Ratio (E/T)." *Gastroenterology* 76:415-17.

Levine, J. 1953. "The Sexual Adjustment of Alcoholics: A Clinical Study of a Selected Sample." *Q. J. Stud. Alcohol* 16:675-80.

Levy, R. I. 1940. "Psychodynamic Functions of Alcohol." *Q. J. Stud. Alcohol* 1:21-44.

Liles, R. E., and D. Childs. 1986. "Similarities in Family Dynamics of Incest and Alcohol Abuse." *Alcohol, Health Res. World* (Fall): 66-69.

Machover, S., F. S. Puzz, K. Machover, and F. Pulumeau. 1959. "Clinical and Objective Studies of Personality Variables in Alcoholism. III: An Objective Study of Homosexuality in Alcoholism." *Q. J. Stud. Alcohol* 20:528-42.

Mandell, W., and C. Miller. 1983. "Male Sexual Dysfunction as Related to Alcohol Consumption: A Pilot Study." *Alcoholism: Clin. Exptl. Res.* 7, no. 1:65-69.

McCaghy, C. H. 1968. "Drinking and Deviance Disavowal: The Case of Child Molesters." *Social Problems* 16:43-49.

McFarland, B., ed. 1984. *Sexuality and Recovery* (Center City, MN: Hazelden Foundation).

Meiselman, K. C. 1978. "Participants in Father-Daughter Incest." In *Incest: A Psychological Study of Causes and Effects, with Treatment Recommendations*, edited by K. C. Meiselman (San Francisco, CA: Jossey-Bass).

Mendelson, J. H., and N. K. Mello. 1974. "Alcohol, Aggression, and Androgens." *Res. Nerv. Ment. Dis.* 52:225-47.

______. 1979. "Biologic Concomitants of Alcoholism." *N. Engl. J. Med.* October 25, pp. 912-21.

Mohr, J. W., R. E. Turner, and M. B. Terry. 1964. *Pedophilia and Exhibitionism* (Toronto: University of Toronto Press).

Moos, R. H., J. W. Finney, and W. Gamble. 1982. "The Process of Recovery from Alcoholism. II: Comparing Spouses of Alcoholic Patients and Matched Community Controls." *J. Stud. Alcohol* 43: 889-909.

Moos, R. H., and B. S. Moos. 1984. "The Process of Recovery from Alcoholism. III: Comparing Functioning in Families of Alcoholics with Matched Control Families." *J. Stud. Alcohol* 45:111-18.

Nardi, P. 1981. "Alcohol Treatment and the Non-Traditional 'Family' Structure of Gays and Lesbians." Presented at the National Council on Alcoholism Forum, New Orleans, April.

______. 1982. "Alcoholism and Homosexuality: A Theoretical Perspective." *J. Homosexuality* 7, no. 4:9-25.

Nichols, F. L., and D. Haines. 1979. "The Difficulties of Dual Denial in the Treatment of Sex Offenders with Alcoholism." *Internat. Offender Ther. Comp. Criminol.* 23:214-20.

Penick, E. C., B. J. Powell, and M. R. Read. 1984. "Sex-Role Affiliation Among Male Alcoholics." *J. Clin. Psychol.* 40:359-63.

Persky, H., K. D. Smith, and G. K. Basu. 1971. "Relation of Psychologic Measures of Aggression and Hostility to Testosterone Production in Man." *Psychosomat. Med.* 33:149.

Phillip, E. 1966. "La personalté des délinquants d'inceste." *Acta Medicinae Legalis Socialis* (Liége) 19:199-201. Cited in Lukianowicz, N., "Incest. I: Paternal Incest." *Br. J. Psychiatr.* 120 (1972):301-13.

Polich, J. M., D. J. Armor, and H. B. Braiker. 1980. "The Course of Alcoholism: Four Years After Treatment." Prepared for the U.S. National Institute on Alcohol Abuse and Alcoholism (Santa Monica, CA: Rand Corporation).

Powell, D. J. 1984. "Treatment of Impotence in Male Alcoholics." In *Alcoholism and Sexual Dysfunction: Issues in Clinical Management*, edited by D. J. Powell (New York: The Haworth Press), pp. 65-82.

Quarantana, J. V. 1947. "Alcoholism: A Study of Emotional Maturity and Homosexuality as Related to Factors in Compulsive Drinking." Thesis, Fordham University, 1947. Quoted in W. McCord and J. McCord, *Origins of Alcoholism* (London: Tavistock, 1960).

Rada, R. T. 1975. "Alcoholism and Forcible Rape." *Am. J. Psychiatr.* 132:444-46.

______. 1976. "Alcoholism and the Child Molester." *Annals N.Y. Acad. Sci.* 273:492-96.

Rada, R. T., D. R. Laws, and R. Kellner. 1976. "Plasma Testosterone Levels in the Rapist." *Psychosomat. Med.* 38:257-68.

Rajan, V., M. Powell, A. Burgett, and V. Bhalla. 1982. "Ethanol-Induced Release of Adenosine-3′5′-Monophosphate into the Medium by Rats Testes *In Vitro*." *Endocrinology* 110:80-88.

Reynolds, L. 1986. Quoted in the *Journal of the Addiction Research Foundation*, October 1, p. 4.

Rose, R. M. P. P. Borden, and D. S. Bernstein. 1972. "Plasma Testosterone in the Male Rhesus: Influences of Sexual and Social Stimuli." *Science* 178:643.

Rose, R. M., J. W. Holady, and D. S. Bernstein. 1971. "Plasma Testosterone, Dominance, Rank and Aggressive Behavior in Rhesus Monkeys." *Nature* 231:366.

Rubin, E., C. S. Lieber, K. Altman, G. Gordon, and H. Southren. 1976. "Prolonged Ethanol Consumption Increases Testosterone Metabolism in the Liver." *Science* 191:563-64.

Sarrel, P., and W. Masters. 1982. "Sexual Molestation of Men by Women." *Arch. Sex. Behav.* 11, no. 2:117-32.

Scheig, R. 1975. "Changes in Sexual Performance Due to Liver Disease." *Med. Aspects Hum. Sex.* 9:67-69.

Scott, E. M. 1977. "The Sexual Offender." *Internat. J. Offender Ther. Comp. Criminol.* 21, no. 3:255-63.

Sherfey, M. J. 1955. "Psychopathology and Character Structure in Chronic Alcoholism." In *Etiology of Chronic Alcoholism*, edited by O. Diethelm (Springfield, IL: Charles C Thomas).

Shirley, C., and K. Shirley. 1981. *The Process of Recovery for the Alcoholic and the Family* (New York: New York City Affiliate, National Council on Alcoholism).

Small, E., and B. Leach. 1977. "Counseling Homosexual Alcoholics." *J. Stud. Alcohol* 38:2077-86.

Southren, A. L., G. G. Gordon, J. Olivo, F. Rafii, and W. S. Rosenthal. 1973. "Androgen Metabolism in Cirrhosis of the Liver." *Metabolism* 22:695-702.

Steinglass, P. 1981. "The Alcoholic Family at Home: Patterns of Interaction in Dry, Wet, and Transitional Stages of Alcoholism." *Arch. Gen. Psychol.* 38:578-84.

Steinglass, P., D. Davis, and D. Berenson. 1977. "Observations of Conjointly Hospitalized 'Alcoholic Couples' During Sobriety and Intoxication: Implications for Theory and Therapy." *Family Process* (Baltimore), vol. 16.

Steinglass, P., S. Weiner, and J. Mendelson. 1971. "Interactional Issues as Determinants of Alcoholism." *Am. J. Psychol.* 128:275-80.

Swanson, D. W. 1968. "Adult Sexual Abuse of Children." *Dis. Nerv. Syst.* 29:677-83.

Tinklenberg, J., and K. M. Woodrow. 1974. "Drug Use Among Youthful Assaultive and Sexual Offenders." *Association for Research in Nervous and Mental Diseases* 52:209-24.

Van Thiel, D. 1977. "Therapy of Sexual Dysfunction in Alcohol Abusers: A Pandora's Box." *Gastroenterology* 72, no. 6:1354-56.

Van Thiel, D., C. F. Cobb, G. B. Herman, H. A. Perez, L. Estes, and J. Gavaler. 1981. "An Examination of Various Mechanisms for Ethanol-Induced Testicular Injury: Studies Utilizing the Isolated Perfused Rat Testes." *Endocrinology* 109:2009-15.

Van Thiel, D., and J. Gavaler. 1985. "Endocrine Effects of Chronic Alcohol Abuse: Hypothalamic-Pituitary-Gonadal Axis." In *Alcohol and the Brain: Chronic Effects*, edited by R. E. Tarter and D. H. Van Thiel (New York: Plenum), pp. 69-79.

Van Thiel, D., and R. Lester. 1974. "Sex and Alcohol." *N. Engl. J. Med.* 291:252-53.

———. 1976. "Sex and Alcohol: A Second Peak." *N. Engl. J. Med.* 29: 835-36.

Virkkunen, M. 1974. "Incest Offences and Alcoholism." *Medicine, Science and the Law* 14:124-28.

Vittek, J., G. G. Gordon, A. Southren, S. Rappaport, P. Munnanji, and C. Lieber. 1981. "Effect of Ethanol Intake on Cellular Regulation of Testosterone 5-Alpha-A-Ring-Reductase in Rat Oral Tissues." *J. Pharmacol. Exp. Ther.* 217:411-15.

Wall, J. H. 1936. "A Study of Alcoholism in Men." *Am. J. Psychiatr.* 92: 1389-1401.

Weinberg, J. 1977. *Sex and Recovery: Straight Talk for the Chemically Dependent and Those They Love* (Minneapolis, MN: Recovery Press).

Westermeyer, J. 1978. "Incest in Psychiatric Practice: A Description of Patients and Incestuous Relationships." *J. Clin. Psychol.* 39:643-48.

Whalley, L. J. 1978. "Sexual Adjustment of Male Alcoholics." *Acta Psychiatr. Scand.* 58:281-98.

Whitfield, C. L. 1980. "Children of Alcoholics: Treatment Issues." *Maryland State Med. J.* 29:86-91.

Williams, K. 1976. "An Overview of Sexual Problems in Alcoholism." Proceedings of a workshop on sexual counseling for persons with alcohol problems." University of Pittsburgh Medical School, October, pp. 1-23.

Wilson, G., D. Lawson, and D. Abrams. 1978. "Effects of Alcohol on Sexual Arousal in Male Alcoholics." *J. Abnorm. Psychol.* 87:609-16.

Wincze, John P., and C. Qualls. 1984. "A Comparison of Structural Patterns of Sexual Arousal in Male and Female Homosexuals." *Archiv. Sex. Behav.* 13, no. 4:361-70.

Zweben, A. 1986. "Problem Drinking and Marital Adjustment." *J. Stud. Alcohol* 47:167-72.

3

The Influence of Alcohol on Sexual Response in Female Social Drinkers

INTRODUCTION

Historically, little research is done on female populations. This pertains not only to mental health research but to medical investigation in general.

The advent of the women's movement, coupled with public awareness of the fetal alcohol syndrome, has contributed to a slight acceleration of interest in alcoholism among women. Simultaneously, the exposition by Masters and Johnson of the specific events that take place during sexual response in the human female have furthered our understanding of female sexuality.

Work on the interaction between alcohol and sex among female social drinkers is relatively sparse. In this chapter, we will review some popular beliefs shared by society and, until recently, by clinical investigators. We will also review more recent psychophysiological studies measuring the effects of varying blood alcohol levels as compared with subjects' expectations about the way in which alcohol will affect their sexual response.

CLINICAL OBSERVATIONS AND CORRELATIONAL INVESTIGATIONS

Popular Beliefs About Alcohol

In the late nineteenth and early twentieth centuries, strict gender roles served to reinforce family stability. Double standards of behavior for men and women applied to sexual conduct and career choices, and to drinking. Although there has been significant change in the past 20 years, alcohol use has generally been considered unladylike (Lender 1985). Divorced and unemployed women have higher rates of consumption, but employed married women have significantly higher rates of alcohol consumption than young single working women or middle-aged unemployed married women (Johnson 1982). This increased consumption among employed married women is thought to result from conflict due to lack of social acceptance for women in nontraditional roles.

In spite of the stigma attached both to drinking and to nontraditional roles, many women believe that alcohol has aphrodisiac qualities. In a study of male and female college students, 70 women, divided equally into groups of heavy and light drinkers, completed sets of questions directly assessing alcohol-related attitudes and behavior. The heavy drinking group scored higher on a sensation-seeking needs scale, with an especially high need for disinhibition. The results suggested that the women in this population drank because they believed alcohol would enhance "social pleasure" (Ratliff and Burkhart 1984).

Zucker, Battistich, and Langer (1981) tested the hypothesis that heavy drinking in women developed because of difficulties in achieving intimacy. They suspected that heavy drinkers would be more sexually active than light drinkers, but that the increased drinking reflected an attempt to ameliorate disturbance and conflict about relationships. Three hundred and seventy unmarried women undergraduates participated in a study of personality and dating patterns. Drinking histories were obtained. Women who reported drinking five or six drinks on all drinking occasions, two to three times per month, and women who drank three or more times per day, consuming one to two drinks each time, were classified as heavy drinkers. Histories were also taken of frequency of sexual intercourse compared with duration of relationship.

Heavy drinkers had earlier onsets of heterosexual experience, more frequent intercourse, and a higher rate of current sexual activity than light drinkers. The first part of the hypothesis, greater sexual activity among heavy drinkers, seemed to be borne out by the data. However, Zucker et al. concluded that there was no support for their assumption that heavy drinkers showed greater sex-role conflict than light drinkers after they had analyzed fantasy measures for the entire population studied. Earlier literature had proclaimed a much more clear-cut relationship between drinking and gender conflict in females (Lolli 1956) as well as males (Jones 1965). There was "slight and equivocal evidence" that traditional sex-role attitudes were connected with infrequent drinking. Differences between nondrinkers and drinkers were somewhat greater than those between heavy and light consumers of alcohol (Zucker, Battistich, and Langer 1981). Lack of support for a direct association between increased drinking and conflicting roles in women was noted also by Parker et al. (1980).

Harvey and Beckman (1986) examined the effects of alcohol consumption on female sexuality and contraceptive use among 69 women, aged 18 to 34. They found that womens' beliefs about the aphrodisiac properties of alcohol did not correspond to daily logs of sexual and drinking activity. The women thought that alcohol enhanced their sexual desire and increased their activity and enjoyment. The logs reflected the reverse. Alcohol consumption was correlated with decreased initiation of sexual activity by the subjects.

Use of alcohol immediately prior to intercourse had no effect on contraceptive use in this population. In contrast, Zucker ete al. (1981: 461) had concluded that heavier alcohol intake was inversely related to the use of contraceptives, despite the lack of a conscious wish to be pregnant.

Women in a nontraditional role were recently compared with their male counterparts in an attempt to correlate drinking patterns and psychosocial measures, such as perceived parental warmth and depressive symptomatology. The population consisted of 107 male and 46 female first-year medical students. Results contradicted the notion that heavier drinking would be associated with greater psychopathology in women. Men and women had similar drinking patterns, although males tended to consume more beer and women more wine. Heavier consumption of alcohol in the female students was correlated with perceptions of parental warmth and low depressive symptomatology. This contrasted weakly with the male population, in which there was a slight tendency for the heavier alcohol consumption to be related inversely to perceptions of parental bonding and directly to depressive symptoms. The authors suggest that drinking in their female population symbolizes successful identification with previously male social roles. They hope that further research will elucidate symbolic meanings attached to drinking by men and women in different occupational and social contexts (Richman and Flaherty 1986).

Although women believe that drinking will increase their sense of being attractive, some data contradict this. Most studies have not included women subjects (Berg 1971; Vanderpool 1969). Studies that report lower self-esteem in alcoholic women as compared with both alcoholic men and nonalcoholic women suggest linkage between low self-esteem and alcoholic consumption but don't tell us whether or not the low self-esteem preceded the age at which drinking began. We are left with no information about the pre-morbid state of the alcoholic women (Konovsky and Wilsnak 1982). We are also uncertain about the effect of social drinking on self-esteem in women.

Konovsky and Wilsnak examined the effect of social drinking in natural settings on self-esteem in married couples. Ninety-two married pairs of men and women between the ages of 19 and 52 were selected from responses to advertisements and bulletin board posters. Only subjects who drank socially were accepted for the study. Those who abstained completely from alcohol as well as problem drinkers were excluded. Couples attended wet and dry parties which were similar except for the availability of alcohol. Couples answered a self-administered questionnaire, the Tennessee Self-Concept Scale, and parts of a sex-typed personality trait measure, the Personal Attributes Questionnaire (PAQ), in a separate session and after the wet or dry party situation to which they were assigned. The parties took place several days to weeks after the initial questionnaire session.

Baseline self-esteem was independent of the subject's gender or party assignment. There was a significant decrease in women's self-esteem scores after drinking. To test the hypothesis that women in traditional sex roles defined drinking as inappropriate, the authors classified the women as having traditional or nontraditional values based on their PAQ scores. There was no difference in scores of women identified as having traditional values versus those having nontraditional values after attending a dry party. After a party session in which alcohol was served, the women designated traditional scored lower then baseline on subscales of Personal Self, Family Self, and Social Self and two summary scales, Identity and Behavior, thus producing lower Total Positive scores. Women who were classified as heavy drinkers based on their consumption at the party did not have significantly lower self-esteem scores than women who were classified as light drinkers. The Personal Self score was more consistently affected by the consumption of alcohol than the other subscales (Konovsky and Wilsnak 1982).

In a balanced placebo design experiment, Abrams and Wilson (1979) tested the effect that expectation of drinking alcohol would have on social anxiety. There had been a widely accepted notion that alcohol serves to disinhibit sexual and aggressive behavior by "neutralizing anxiety reactions" which would be otherwise present. Alcohol's alleged effect on tension reduction has been assumed to be a motivation for drinking. The Abrams and Wilson experiment contradicted this. Subjects' self-reports indicated that they expected their anxiety to be lowered by alcohol and thought it had been lowered when they believed they had consumed an alcoholic beverage, but objective measures indicated an opposite effect. Groups who expected alcohol, whether they received alcohol or placebo, had significantly elevated physiological measures of arousal, including heart rate and skin conductance. In addition, after finishing their drinks, subjects were asked to interact with a male confederate of the experimenter. Measures of social interaction confirmed increased rather than decreased social discomfort in the subjects who believed they drank alcohol as compared with subjects who believed they drank a nonalcoholic beverage, regardless of the actual drink content.

Since the 1960s there has been an upward surge of 17 points in the percentage of women in the population who drink. A Gallup survey in 1939 showed that 70 percent of men used alcoholic beverages compared with 45 percent of women. The figures now indicate little difference between 1939 and 1986 in the number of male drinkers; 75 percent of the male population drink. The percentage of women who drink is 62. Among teenagers interviewed in a national Gallup pole, 39 percent of the adolescent boys drink alcohol as compared with 38 percent of adolescent girls. In the college student population, 75 percent of the males consume alcohol, as do 69 percent of the females. This suggests a trans-generational closing of the drinking gap between men and women.

There does seem to be a lingering difference between the sexes in attitudes about drinking. Fifty-nine percent of teenage girls think that teenagers who are regular alcohol consumers will have problems in adult life, compared with 46 percent of teenage boys who share this opinion. Twenty-one percent of adult women favor a return of Prohibition, as compared with 12 percent of adult men. Women questioned in the most recent Gallup pole emphasized social reasons for drinking, while men cited personal enjoyment as their primary motivation. Women showed greater concern than men over the effect of alcohol abuse on the family and society. They were also more willing than men to vote for strong measures to combat drunk driving and other alcohol-related dangers (Gallup 1986).

Relationship of Sex Victimization to Intoxicated State of Female Victims

Women tend to believe that drinking alcohol will make them more vulnerable sexually (Konovsky and Wilsnak 1982; Abrams and Wilson 1979). There are statistics that would indicate some foundation for this anxiety (Amir 1967; Johnson, Gibson, and Linden, 1978). In Amir's study, women who were drunk or merely drinking in public places were more vulnerable to rape. Violent rape was performed less often when only the victim was drinking; force was used most often when both the victim and the rapist were drinking (Johnson, Gibson, and Linden 1978).

Barling and Bolan (1981), using a balanced placebo design, studied the interaction of alcohol with locus of control in 19 male and female college students. Women seemed to have a more external locus of control after the use of alcohol than before, as contrasted with males. Those women who were given the experimental instruction to expect alcohol, and who received alcohol as opposed to placebo, perceived their behavior to be controlled externally, by environmental events. Men under the same experimental condition, perceived that their individual inner controls determined external events. The men thought that they controlled the world and the women thought that the world controlled them. This is a small study sample, but it would tend to support the notion of increased sexual vulnerability associated with alcohol use.

Filmore (1985), in a survey of 1,395 randomly selected adults, aged 18 and older, found that female victims of sexual crimes resembled a population of problem drinkers. Heavy and frequent drinking increased the risk of sex victimization, especially among women who were young, single, and of low socioeconomic status. Drinking with relatives increased the risk for women. Women were two times as likely to be raped if with someone who was drinking, even if the women themselves were not drinking.

Relative Sparseness of Clinical Observations or Correlational Investigation of Effect of Alcohol on Sexual Response of Female as Compared with Male Social Drinkers

"Most experts comment on human sexual behavior and alcohol as though only males drink and have sexual interests" (Carpenter and Armenti 1971: 521). No reference is made to effects of alcohol in the report by Kinsey et al. (1953) on sexual behavior in the human female. Adverse effects of alcohol on female sexuality are not mentioned by Masters and Johnson (1966) and are only barely alluded to by Kaplan (1974).

One of the barriers to inclusion of women in studies of the effects of alcohol has been doubt about the interaction between blood alcohol levels and phases of the menstrual cycle. Harvey and Beckman reported that frequency of alcohol use did not vary according to menstrual cyclic timing, but that the quantity of alcohol consumed was higher in the luteal phase (Harvey and Beckman 1985). Differences in alcohol pharmacokinetics as a function of menstrual phase were also unconfirmed by Hay et al. (1984). Brick et al. (1986) suggest that previous studies, which had indicated that hormonal differences may explain why women reach higher BALs at a faster rate than men, "may have resulted from the practice of dosing subjects by total body weight rather than by body water weight." In their study of 10 women in their early twenties, the pharmacokinetics and behavioral effects of alcohol were not influenced by menstrual cycle phase. This suggests that research including women can be conducted reliably (Brick et al. 1986).

PSYCHOPHYSIOLOGICAL STUDIES: EFFECT OF ALCOHOL ON VAGINAL BLOOD VOLUME AND PULSE PRESSURE AS MEASURED BY THE VAGINAL PHOTOPLETHYSMOGRAPH

A number of variables affect orgasmic response in women. These have to be taken into account in evaluating the validity of any data regarding the physiological sexual effects of alcohol.

In questionnaire studies there have been differing self-reports of body location for orgasmic experience (Sholty et al. 1984). Stock and Geer (1982) have studied 45 female subjects with a median age of 21. Capacity for sexual fantasy outside of the laboratory and intensity of orgasm in response to a tape, as measured by the vaginal plethysmograph, were directly correlated. In a self-report questionnaire study, orgasmic responsivity in 138 undergraduate women was positively correlated to noncoital heterosexual satisfaction, gratification from masturbation, and comfort with heterosexual contact (Meyers et al. 1983).

A recent study suggests that there is variability between groups of women in duration of orgasm and frequency of contractions and that some women may experience a type of orgasm in which no regular contractions can be detected; 11 nulliparous women manually self-stimulated to orgasm on three separate occasions. Pelvic contraction pressure was measured using vaginal and anal probes simultaneously. Three of the women had orgasms consisting of a series of regular contractions in all three experiments (orgasm type I). Six women always experienced additional irregular contractions after the series of regular contractions (type II). Both types I and II had been noted in men. The type II group had orgasms lasting four times longer than the type I group (50.6 seconds compared with 13.1 seconds). A type III contraction pattern, consisting of a divided regular series, noted previously in man, was not recorded in this experiment. Type IV, previously not found in men, which did not consist of regular contractions, and which lasted a length of time intermediate between I and II, was noted in two of the subjects (Bohlen et al. 1982).

This variability in orgasmic response needs to be kept in mind when we evaluate the physiological effect of alcohol on female sexuality in the works of Malatesta et al. (1982) and Wilson and Lawson (1976, 1978).

Malatesta et al. (1982), using a repeated measures design with monthly experimental sessions, tested the hypothesis that increasing levels of alcohol intoxication were related to symptomatic changes in female orgasmic experience. Eighteen university women were sustained at four different blood alcohol levels in counterbalanced order prior to watching sexually explicit videotapes and engaging in masturbation to orgasm. The vaginal photoplethysmograph, complemented with a behavioral latency measure, indicated a progressive decrease in vaginal engorgement and an increase in orgasmic latency with increasing blood alcohol concentrations. Paradoxically, women reported a subjective increase in orgasmic response and pleasure under conditions of moderate to high intoxication. The authors suggest that women who have alcohol-related orgasmic dysfunction will show improvement if they are alcohol-free. They expect that, in normal women, modest intake of alcohol will result in greater feelings of arousal, enhanced orgasm, and only a slight delay in the time it takes to reach orgasm.

Wilson and Lawson (1976) gave 16 university women four doses of alcohol of differing potency in counterbalanced order. The BALs achieved were 0 mg percent, 25 mg percent, 50 mg percent, and 75 mg percent. Half of the women were given the expectancy instruction that higher doses of alcohol would increase their sexual response and half were told that higher doses would decrease response. Women in each of the four weekly sessions were shown an erotic film, a nonerotic film, and one of four different TAT cards per session. Wilson and Lawson believed that vaginal pulse pressure is the most reliable measure of sexual response in women. Physiological responses to the film were measured by vaginal plethysmograph, along with EMG recordings of frontalis muscular tension. Women were asked to predict their response to erotic stimuli. They predicted enhanced stimulation with alcohol regardless of instructional set. Subjects were each given a second questionnaire during the erotic film in which they were to estimate their degree of intoxication and the effect that alcohol was having on their sexual arousal. Self-reports indicated perceived increased arousal with increasing doses of alcohol. This was in direct contrast to physiological measures, which showed a direct linear negative effect of alcohol on vaginal pulse pressure. EMG recordings did not correlate with arousal. Sexual content in response to the TAT cards was unaffected by "alcohol levels, sessions, or instructional set. Nor was there a significant correlation between this measure and vaginal pressure pulse scores."

The results replicate the findings of Farkas and Rosen (1976) and Briddell and Wilson (1976) with male subjects, in which increasing intoxication produced a progressive reduction in sexual arousal in response to visual erotic stimulation (see Chapter 1). Unlike men, women did not seem able to estimate their own physiological responses accurately; they consistently perceived themselves to be experiencing increased arousal as they became more intoxicated. Perhaps this is because male sexual arousal or its lack is more obvious visually. Henson and Rubin (1971) have demonstrated that men can inhibit tumescence voluntarily or facilitate it in response to visual erotic stimuli. This suggests cognitive mediation of sexual response.

In a further experiment (Wilson and Lawson 1978) 40 university women, aged 18 to 35, were assigned randomly to a 2 × 2 balanced placebo design study. Half of the women were told to expect that they were going to drink a beverage containing alcohol and half were told that their beverage would contain tonic only. The women were assigned to one of four experimental condition groups, consisting of expect alcohol-receive alcohol, expect alcohol-receive tonic, expect tonic-receive tonic, expect tonic-receive alcohol. Subjects were then given their drinks, attaining a pre-film viewing BAL of 35 mg percent or 0 mg percent, depending on beverage content. Following this they viewed one nonerotic film and two erotic films, one explicitly heterosexual and one explicitly homosexual. Vaginal pressure pulse was measured by means of a vaginal photoplethysmograph during the film viewing. Regardless of expectation concerning drink content, the groups who actually drank alcohol showed significantly decreased sexual arousal in response to the heterosexual film. Ninety percent of the women who expected and received tonic only and 87 percent of the remaining groups predicted increased arousal to the heterosexual film. For the homosexual film, 45 percent in the two expect-alcohol groups and 50 percent in the expect-tonic groups predicted increased arousal. In contrast to the heterosexual film, no significant effect of alcohol was detected in the homosexual film. The authors note that the film order wasn't counterbalanced and suggest the possibility that the BAL during the homosexual film wasn't high enough to impair sexual response. The BAL at the end of the film sequence was 22 mg percent. The homosexual film was always shown last.

In Wilson and Lawson's balanced placebo design experiment with male social drinkers, expectancy enhanced arousal. Men who expected to receive alcohol showed increased penile tumescence regardless of actual beverage content. In contrast, with women, alcohol decreased sexual response but expectancy had no effect. This was in spite of the fact that the BAL in the experiment using male subjects was slightly higher, at 40 mg percent (Wilson and Lawson 1976).

SUMMARY

Many factors influence sexual response to alcohol among female social drinkers. On one hand, inebriated women are never acceptable in our society. There are situations among men where intoxication is sanctioned: fraternity parties, bachelor parties, a night out with the boys. I can think of no situational counterpart for women. For both men and women, increased sexual risk-taking is supposed to accompany drinking. In the data reviewed in this chapter, women sense that such behavioral loosening up will result in social disapproval and increase their vulnerability to sexual attack.

On the other hand, the data suggest that women expect that alcohol will enhance their sexual desire and performance and even experience this subjectively, although actual measurements of vaginal pulse pressure and orgasmic latency in response to erotic stimuli are directly contrary to expectation. Women are therefore inaccurate estimators. The true effects of alcohol on sexuality in female social drinkers are all negative. Women predict that alcohol will make them more at ease socially, and enhance their sexual performance; actually, the expectation of drinking alcohol increases social anxiety and the presence of alcohol diminishes orgasmic capacity.

More recent studies correlating self-esteem in nontraditional roles with drinking seem to disprove the notion that women with career aspirations suffer from insecurity as a consequence of role conflict and therefore use alcohol as an anesthetic. Drinking appears to be accepted by these women as congruent with their self-image. It is possible that if expectation of drinking were to be correlated with social anxiety in this group, the results would differ from those in the study by Abrams and Wilson (1979).

The sparseness of physiological data available about women's sexual response at pharmacologically effective BALs has to do with concern about the influence of menstrual cycle phases. More recent studies fail to confirm that hormonal variations in women affect the influence of alcohol on certain behaviors and suggest that exclusion of women from experiments on those grounds may not be warranted.

Another reason for exclusion of women from alcohol studies has been social rejection of the notion that women drink. Although inebriated women are not socially acceptable, the gap between numbers of male and female social drinkers is closing. This will provide researchers with a larger sample to draw upon.

REFERENCES

Abrams, D., and G. T. Wilson. 1979. "Effects of Alcohol on Social Anxiety in Women: Cognitive vs. Physiological Processes." *J. Abnorm. Psychol.* 88, no. 2:161-73.

Amir, M. 1967. "Alcohol and Forcible Rape." *Br. J. Addict.* 62:219-32.

Barling, J., and K. Bolan. 1981. "Effects of Alcohol Expectancies, Sex and Social Setting on Locus of Control." *J. Stud. Alcohol* 42, no. 7:680-84.

Berg, N. L. 1971. "Effects of Alcohol Intoxication on Self-Concept." *Q. J. Stud. Alcohol* 32:442-53.

Bohlen, J. G., J. Held, M. O. Sanderson, and A. Ahlgren. 1982. "The Female Orgasm: Pelvic Contractions." *Arch. Sex. Behav.* 11, no. 5: 367-86.

Brick, J., P. E. Nathan, M. S. Westrick, W. Frankenstein, and A. Shapiro. 1986. "The Effect of Menstrual Cycle on Blood Alcohol Levels and Behavior." *J. Stud. Alcohol* 47, no. 6:472-77.

Briddell, D. W., and G. T. Wilson. 1976. "The Effects of Alcohol and Expectancy Set on Male Sexual Arousal." *J. Abnorm. Psychol.* 85: 225-34.

Carpenter, J. A., and N. P. Armenti. 1971. "Some Effects of Ethanol on Human Sexual and Aggressive Behavior." In *The Biology of Alcoholism*, vol. 2, edited by B. Kissen and H. Begleiter (New York: Plenum Press), pp. 509-43.

Farkas, G. M., and R. C. Rosen. 1976. "Effect of Alcohol on Elicited Male Sexual Response." *J. Stud. Alcohol* 37, no. 3:265-72.

Filmore, K. M. 1985. "Social Victims of Drinking." *Br. J. Addict.* 80: 307-14.

Gallant, D. M. 1986. "A Study of the Victims of Alcohol Abusers." *Alcoholism: Clin. Exptl. Res.* 10, no. 3:358-59.

Gallup, G. 1986. "Women: A Powerful Force for Moderation." *Alcoholism Addict.* (November-December):13.

Harvey, S. M., and L. J. Beckman. 1985. "Cyclic Fluctuations in Alcohol Consumption Among Female Social Drinkers." *Alcoholism: Clin. Exptl. Res.* 9, no. 5:465-67.

______. 1986. "Alcohol Consumption, Female Sexual Behavior and Contraceptive Use." *J. Stud. Alcohol* 47, no. 4:327-32.

Hay, W. M., P. E. Nathan, H. W. Heermans, and W. Frankenstein. 1984. "Menstrual Cycle, Tolerance and Blood Alcohol Level Discrimination Ability." *Addict. Behav.* 9:67-77.

Henson, D. E., and H. B. Rubin. 1971. "Voluntary Control of Eroticism." *J. Appl. Behav. Anal.* 4:37-44.

Johnson, P. B. 1982. "Sex Differences, Women's Roles and Alcohol Use: Preliminary National Data." *J. Soc. Issues* 38, no. 2:93-116.

Johnson, S. D., L. Gibson, and R. Linden. 1978. "Alcohol and Rape in Winnepeg, 1966-75." *J. Stud. Alcohol* 39:1887-94.

Jones, B. M., and M. R. Jones. 1976. "Women and Alcohol: Intoxication, Metabolism, and the Menstrual Cycle." In *Alcoholism Problems in Women and Children*, edited by M. Greenblatt and M. A. Schuckit (New York: Grune and Stratton).

Jones, M. C. 1965. "Personality Correlates and Antecedents of Drinking Pattern in Adult Males." *J. Consult. Clin. Psychol.* 1:441-52.

Kaplan, H. 1974. *The New Sex Therapy* (New York: Brunner/Mazel).

Kinsey, A., W. Pomeroy, C. Martin, and P. Gebhard. 1953. *Sexual Behavior in the Human Female* (Philadelphia, PA: Saunders).

Konovsky, M., and S. C. Wilsnak. 1982. "Social Drinking and Self-Esteem in Married Couples." *J. Stud. Alcohol* 43, no 3:319-33.

Lender, M. 1985. "A Special Stigma: Women and Alcoholism in the Late 19th and Early 20th Centuries." In *Alcohol Interventions: Historical and Sociocultural Approaches*, edited by Strug, Piryadarsima, and Heyman (New York, London: The Haworth Press), pp. 41-57.

Lolli, G. 1956. "Alcoholism as a Disorder of the Love Disposition." *Q. J. Stud. Alcohol* 17:96-107.

Malatesta, V. J., R. H. Pollack, T. D. Crotty, and L. J. Peacock. 1982. "Acute Alcohol Intoxication and Female Orgasmic Response." *J. Sex Res.* 18:1-17.

Masters, W. H., and V. E. Johnson. 1966. *Human Sexual Response* (Boston, MA: Little, Brown).

Meyers, de R., Jr., P. Kilmann, R. Wanglass, and A. Stout. 1983. "Dimensions of Female Sexuality: A Factor Analysis." *Arch. Sex. Behav.* 12, no 2:159-66.

Parker, D. A., E. S. Parker, M. W. Wolz, and T. C. Harford. 1980. "Sex Roles and Alcohol Consumption: A Research Note." *J. Health Soc. Behav.* 21:43-48.

Ratliff, K. G., and B. R. Burkhart. 1984. "Sex Differences in Motivations for and Effects of Drinking Among College Students." *J. Stud. Alcohol* 45, no. 1:26-32.

Richman, J. A., and J. A. Flaherty. 1986. "Sex Differences in Drinking Among Medical Students: Patterns and Psychosocial Correlates." *J. Stud. Alcohol* 47, no. 4:283-89.

Sholty, M. J., P. Ephross, S. M. Plaut, S. H. Fischman, J. F. Charnas, and C. A. Cody. 1984. "Female Orgasmic Experience: A Subjective Study." *Arch. Sex. Behav.* 13, no. 2:155-64.

Stock, W. E., and J. H. Geer. 1982. "A Study of Fantasy-Based Sexual Arousal in Women." *Arch. Sex. Behav.* 11, no. 1:33-48.

Vanderpool, J. A. 1969. "Alcoholism and the Self-Concept." *Q. J. Stud. Alcohol* 30:59-77.

Wilson, G. T., and D. M. Lawson. 1976. "The Effect of Alcohol on Sexual Arousal in Women." *J. Abnorm. Psychol.* 85, no. 3:489-97.

______. 1978. "Expectancies, Alcohol and Sexual Arousal in Women." *J. Abnorm. Psychol.* 87, no. 3:358-67.

Zucker, R. A., V. A. Battistich, and G. B. Langer. 1981. "Sexual Behavior, Sex-Role Adaptation and Drinking in Young Women." *J. Stud. Alcohol* 42, no. 5:457-65.

4

Sexual Response in Female Alcoholics

INTRODUCTION

Complexity permeates most areas of investigation regarding alcoholism in women. Until recently, the population of female alcoholics was considered too small for statistically significant observations to be made. Because of double standards for men and women in regard to drinking (Blume 1986; Lender 1985), alcoholism in women has been viewed harshly. Prevalence may have been underreported as a consequence of "closet" or solitary drinking on the part of women (Heath 1986). It is also possible that there is a true increase in the incidence of alcoholism in women since World War II (Blume 1986). Treatment centers differ widely in their estimations of the number of women in their alcoholic populations. However, women alcoholics are now thought to exist in numbers sufficient for the development of programs specifically tailored to their needs.

It has been postulated that affective disorder occurs in female alcoholics more often than in males (Hesselbrock, Meyer, and Keener 1985). Antecedents such as parental rejection or abuse are thought to produce increased sexual inhibition in female alcoholics who then use alcohol for its alleged aphrodisiac properties. As noted in the last chapter, Wilson and Lawson (1976, 1978; and Malatesta et al. 1982) demonstrated actual decrease in sexual arousal in women who had elevated blood alcohol levels. Popular beliefs about alcohol were thus negated by physiological evidence (see Chapter 3).

Although sons of alcoholic fathers are thought to have a fourfold greater chance of developing alcoholism than men in the general population (Goodwin 1985), only one study seems to have considered maternal genetic transmission for women. Bohman, Sigvardsson, and Cloninger (1981) examined the occurrence of alcohol abuse in 913 Swedish daughters adopted by nonrelatives at an early age. There was a threefold increase in the incidence of alcohol abuse among daughters whose biologic mothers were alcoholic. Daughters of alcoholic fathers did not have a significant increase in the incidence of alcohol abuse. Alcoholism on the part of adoptive parents did not increase the incidence of alcoholism in their adopted daughters.

The long-term hormonal effects of alcohol produce sexual dysfunction in male alcoholics. The hormonal effects in females are suspected but sufficient research has not yet been done. Hormonal effects, if present, can account for decreased sexual desire and anorgasmia even without the contribution of antecedent psychological or sociocultural factors.

Relationships in families in which the wife is an active alcoholic are most often deeply affected not only because of sexual dysfunction as a result of psychopathology and/or hormonal changes but also because of behavioral deterioration. Husbands and children develop a reciprocal reaction pattern to unpredictable moodiness, explosions of temper, emotional neglect, inattention to housekeeping chores, and deterioration in appearance. Rehabilitation programs must involve the family in treatment whenever possible.

Recovery for single heterosexual women is influenced by a variety of factors including age, employment status, support network, live-in relationships, and coexisting psychiatric illnesses, if present. Rehabilitated lesbian alcoholics must contend with all of the above as well as the triple social stigma of being homosexual, female, and alcoholic.

HORMONAL CHANGES

Menstrual cycle irregularities among female alcoholics have been observed by clinicians since the nineteenth century (Abel 1985). In spite of this there are few studies that directly monitor gonadal functioning in alcoholic women (Hill 1984). Hugues et al. (1978) studied hypothalamic-pituitary-gonadal functioning in 11 alcoholic women who were menopausal. They found subgroups of post-menopausal women and women in menopausal transition. Estradiol, FSH, and prolactin levels were measured at baseline and after LHRH and TRH administration. The only notable difference between the alcoholic women and a control group of similar age was that plasma estradiol was somewhat lower in alcoholic women following administration of both LHRH and FSH. Gavaler (1985) commented that alcohol use or misuse "has received no attention as a factor or as a variable to be controlled in studies evaluating determinants of estrogen levels in post-menopausal non-alcoholic women."

Animals whose ovaries were removed were found to have increased estrogen levels following ethanol administration. Obviously, the source of the estrogen was extra-ovarian. If alcohol increases extra-ovarian production of estrogen, it is thought possible that post-menopausal women might "self-medicate" menopausal symptoms with alcohol (Mendelson 1986).

Investigations of the effect of alcohol on hormonal levels of non-menopausal normal women, conducted by Mendelson, Mello, and Ellingboe (1981), yielded no significant differences in levels of LH and estradiol when alcohol was administered as compared with placebo. Six subjects were given alcohol to achieve blood alcohol levels of 88 mg per 100 ml during days 8, 9, and 10 of one menstrual cycle and placebo during the same days in the following cycle. Prolactin was elevated slightly during the descending portion of the blood alcohol curve.

Alcohol-fed rats developed atrophic ovaries as compared with age-matched rats fed a similar diet with dextrimaltose substituted isocalorically for ethanol (Van Thiel, Gavaler, and Lester 1977).

In rhesus monkeys, alcohol in high doses appears to have a selective effect on the pituitary. LH secretion is unaltered but FSH secretion is suppressed (Mendelson 1986).

Since it is known that exogenous estrogen administration may cause fetal abnormalities (for example, in children of mothers given diethystilbesterol during pregnancy), the role of alcohol in modifying estrogen metabolism in early pregnancy is being investigated in reference to the possible mechanism by which alcohol causes Fetal Alcohol Syndrome. Alcohol requires the cofactor NAD, along with the enzymes alcohol dehydrogenase and aldehyde dehydrogenase in order for ethanol metabolism to take place in the liver. Intrahepatic conversion of the gonadal steroids estrone and estradiol also requires NAD, along with the enzyme 17-beta-steroid-oxireductase. If alcohol competes for NAD as a cofactor for hydrogen transport with these steroids, this would produce increased NADH as compared with NAD. This would shift estrogen metabolism from oxidative to reductive pathways and bring about increased plasma levels of 17-beta-estradiol. Studies are in progress to determine if women who are administered gonadotropin along with ethanol have elevated levels of estradiol. Rhesus monkeys in which a gonadotropin state is induced which is analogous to early pregnancy are being studied during acute and chronic administration of ethanol to see if this stimulates increased estradiol levels (Mendelson 1986).

The cause of premenstrual tension is not clear. Clinical studies have suggested linkage between increased abuse of alcohol and increased dysphoria during the luteal phase of the cycle. No one is sure which comes first, tension inducing increased ethanol intake or an increase in tension induced by increased drinking (Mendelson 1986; Abel 1985).

Decreased Sexual Desire

A lack of interest in sex has been considered characteristic of most female alcoholics. This is attributed to antecedent stresses such as having been brought up in dysfunctional families with cold, domineering, rejecting mothers.

Browne-Mayers, Seelye, and Sillman (1976) interviewed 62 women admitted to the alcohol service at Cornell-Westchester Division from 1968 to 1972. More than 50 percent had had some college education and 20 were high achievers. Twenty-eight reported "inadequate sexual response" due to uncertainty over their sex role. The authors think that ambiguity is the social message given women about their role. They state that women are taught to be sexy but also that interest in sex is improper. They are educated but told that intelligence is unappealing. Working for a living is admirable, but being dependent is feminine.

Lolli (1961) states that women use alcohol to achieve desired sexual responsiveness which they are too inhibited to experience when not drinking, but this in turn renders them vulnerable to sexual attack.

Covington (1986) states that 64 percent of 35 alcoholic women in a recovery program had diminished sexual desire as compared with matched controls. She believes that there is some correlation with sexual dysfunctioning and the experience of incest in childhood. Seventy-four percent of a sample of alcoholic women had experienced sexual abuse, 52 percent physical abuse, and 72 percent emotional abuse. Although 50 percent of her matched controls experienced sexual abuse, she claims a difference for alcoholic women in quantity, quality, and extent of abuse (Covington 1986).

Curran (1937) reported an increase in the number of women alcoholics admitted to Bellevue Hospital between 1931 and 1935. He said that the female population had increased from 1,200 to 1,370 as compared with 7,506 males for the same period. He interviewed 50 women from this sample either because he could analyze the content of their hallucinations or because they had had multiple admissions because of alcoholism. The sexual content of the hallucinations was heterosexual accusations. The voices threatened punishment of sexual activity by mutilation or removal of sexual organs. The majority said that alcohol made them less shy and reserved. He concluded that alcoholic women were narcissistic, attached to their mothers, and threatened by heterosexual behavior. Sixteen women in his sample said they were "frigid." Twenty women among the 50 interviewed reported satisfaction in heterosexual life.

Forrest (1983) also attributes motivation for alcohol abuse to "frigidity" in women.

Apter-Marsh (1984) studied 61 white, heterosexual, middle-class and "reasonably well-educated" alcoholic women, with a mean age of 40 and a mean length of 4.2 years of sobriety. She concluded that sexual adjustment was a function of the point in a woman's drinking career at which she was interviewed. Sex with partners was highest during the active drinking period, with a frequency of 2.2 times per week. It was lower during abstinence (1.3 times per week), but not as low later in sobriety as during the initial abstinence from drinking period, which was 1.1 times per week. Furthermore, Apter-Marsh found that women were able to experience nocturnal sex dreams to the point of orgasm more often than in Kinsey's (1953) frequently cited report. Kinsey had stated that masturbation and sex dreams to the point of orgasm were the best indicators of a female's intrinsic sexuality. Sixty-two percent of women reported these dreams in Apter-Marsh's sample as compared with 20 percent in Kinsey's group. Fifty-one percent of Apter-Marsh's sample enjoyed these dreams during a fully sober period of their lives.

While most authors conclude that alcoholic women suffer from lack of sexual desire, which these writers attribute to role conflict resulting from societal pressures and childhood experience, Apter-Marsh's findings suggest that alcoholic women may have as much interest in sex as nonalcoholic women do. Previous studies had been with populations at rehabilitation centers, days to weeks after drinking had stopped. Apter-Marsh's population had diminished sexual desire in early stages of recovery but regained their desire later. It is possible that findings would have been similar in the other studies cited if the women had been followed through later stages of sobriety.

Anorgasmia

Apter-Marsh stated that, although women were involved in sex with a partner more often while actively drinking, their ability to reach orgasm during this period was greatly reduced. Prior to active drinking, the subjects reported orgasm with partners 36 percent of the time. During active drinking and the early phase of sobriety, orgasm occurred 47 to 48 percent of the time, but in late sobriety it occurred 60 percent of the times that they were engaged in sex with partners. Again this suggests that earlier investigations such as those of Browne-Mayers et al. and Curran, using populations of women who were hospitalized for treatment of alcoholism, have produced findings related to the new and painful separation from alcohol which would have been different had the subjects been interviewed later in the recovery process.

Increased Sexual Inhibition—Less Sexual Activity

Mandel and North (1982) report that 40 percent of their sample of 44 alcoholic women interviewed at a substance abuse clinic had experienced incest. They stress that this percentage is equal to eight times the prevalence in the general population. Furthermore, another 40 percent had experienced rape, four times the general population. This data is supported by Covington (1986), who found that 74 percent of her alcoholic population had been sexually abused as compared with 50 percent of her matched controls. Pinhas (1980) found a large portion of her 34 alcoholic women scored high on a sex-guilt measure as compared with 34 matched controls. Most of her sample were Catholics. She recommends sex education for women in rehabilitation centers so that alcohol will not continue to be used as an anesthetic for guilt. Similar observations about sex guilt were made by Sandmaier (1980). Murphy et al. (1980) reported that 50 percent of a sample of 74 alcoholic women had been sexually abused. Mandel and North found that their sexually abused subpopulation felt "bad" or "nothing" during sex. These women reacted either by never feeling feminine enough and described themselves as passive in bed. Having had a hysterectomy or awareness of sexual problems further threatened their sense of femininity. Another group had rejected femininity as pre-teens. This group was particularly characterized by a history of childhood incest or abuse, often perpetrated by an alcoholic parent. In contrast, Murphy found a lower rate of sexual dysfunction than "previously cited." Only 15 percent complained of low arousal, vaginismus, or dyspareunia. Twenty-eight percent reached orgasm less than 50 percent of the time and 15 percent attained orgasm less than 10 percent of the time. The authors suggest that their questioning may have been more careful and explicit than in earlier studies. They advocate standardized criteria for quantifying the extent and severity of sexual dysfunction among alcoholic women. Benward and Denson-Gerber (1975) and Cohen and Denson-Gerber (1982) found that 44 percent and 33 percent of their substance abuse population, respectively, had been sexually molested as children. Rohsenow, Corbet, and Devine (1986) observed that a prior history of sexual abuse was noted 8 percent of the time when the question was not asked routinely of patients in their substance-abuse treatment program. As soon as the question was asked systematically, the percentage rose to 33 percent. The clinical implication of this is that the incidence of a pre-morbid history of sexual dysfunction among alcoholic women is debatable. However, for those women who experienced childhood sexual abuse, increased sexual inhibition prior to the onset of alcoholism is common. There is growing recognition of the post-traumatic neurosis from which victims of childhood sexual abuse suffer, nonalcoholics as well as alcoholics, and men as well as women. However, debate about the harmfulness of incest continues (Finklehor 1980; Henderson 1983; Gelinas 1983; Orme and Rimmer 1981). Herman, Russell, and Trocki (1986) studied two groups of adult women with histories of incest, a community sample (n = 152), and a group of women who were patients in an outpatient clinic (n = 53). These women were not described as alcoholic. Almost all the women said that they had been upset at the time of the event. Recovery depended on the nature of the sexual abuse experience. Except for a small minority, victims of forceful or repeated and prolonged abuse were unable to escape long-term sequelae. This was especially true if the perpetrators were their fathers or stepfathers. Types of sequelae ranged from negative feelings about men, sex, and themselves, failure to achieve intimacy, and sexual problems, to generalized anxiety. The authors conclude that incest in childhood has a broad range of long-term effects. However, as they point out, women who were so severely traumatized that they were dysfunctional in the community were not included in the nonclinic population.

That most adult victims of rape experience a threat to their sense of body integrity and sexuality seems more generally accepted (Rose 1986). Since intoxication increases the vulnerability of women to sexual attack (Filmore 1985; Gallant 1986; Amir 1967; Johnson, Gibson, and Linden 1978), female alcoholic patients should be asked routinely about whether or not they have been raped. Chronic feelings of rage, distrust, and low self-esteem have accompanied these experiences and may hinder the process of recovery. Often the therapist who asks for this history is the only person with whom they have ever discussed it. Some clinicians are of the opinion that, in a mixed group, male patients or group leaders would be distrusted and that issues such as sexual abuse can be worked on successfully in womens' groups only (Underhill 1986).

Case Histories

Case 1. Beth had a bitter relationship with her husband, marked by previous attempts at marriage counseling, and discussions about the pros and cons of divorce. Intervention dealing explicitly with alcoholism had not occurred before this hospitalization. She had two daughters and two sons, but was troubled by her inability to have tender feelings for them.

Her father, who was an alcoholic, beat her when he was drunk and forced her to have intercourse with him on many occasions when she was aged 12 to 16. Her mother accused her of lying when she asked her for help. Beth continues to believe with apparent justification that her parents had no interest whatsoever in her welfare.

She had very low self-esteem in spite of a graduate degree in literature and employment on the faculty of a university.

She knew that she was desirable to her husband sexually, but berated herself for her lack of interest in sex. Alcohol made it possible for her to be friendlier to him but did nothing to relieve her sexual dysfunction. When intoxicated, she either passed out or stormed out of the house after a loud fight.

Treatment was difficult because of Beth's reflexive distrust of the staff. Gradually she became convinced that alcohol intensified all of her other problems. She also developed a slight degree of bonding to fellow patients who were adult children of alcoholics. A year after being discharged, she still experiences and participates in intense family arguments. She and her husband are once again in marital therapy. For the first time she is hopeful that treatment will work eventually. She trusts her therapist, who is a man. In addition, the points she makes during arguments have credibility, because she is sober when she makes them. Because of increasing positive identification with other women who are successfully recovering from alcoholism, her self-esteem has increased too.

Beth's 18-year-old daughter has been treated for alcohol abuse and has become involved in Al-Anon and AA. Her eldest son is working in the Southwest and seems to be the most well adjusted. The two remaining children are each involved in individual psychotherapy because of academic difficulties in school and behavioral problems at home.

Beth's sexual desire is still lacking. Because her relationship with her husband is so deeply rooted in her childhood experience, it would be reasonable to hope that emerging ability to trust him would gradually facilitate affection. At that point her sexual interest in him might improve.

Case 2. There was a childlike, innocent quality to Margaret's presentation. She was 30, but appeared 15 years younger. She casually mentioned that she had been raped when intoxicated on numerous occasions. She went to bars in neighborhoods away from her home and hitched rides when the bars closed. Rape was deserved, Margaret thought, because, after all, she was an alcoholic. When sober, Margaret didn't want to be touched by anyone and flinched if a patient or staff member of either gender came within two feet of her.

She said that she felt permanently contaminated and hopeless. Her heterosexual adjustment prior to the onset of alcoholism was hard to assess because Margaret had been suspended from private schools four times since the age of 14 for drinking. She had never had a boyfriend and could not picture herself attached to anyone. Her parents were supportive and wanted to help, but Margaret was angry at them for continuing to forgive her.

The first goal of treatment was for Margaret to accept her alcoholism as a disease rather than a character defect. This was attempted through educational films about substance abuse, group discussions, attendance at AA meetings, and individual and group therapy. Margaret felt most comfortable in a women's discussion group because several group members revealed that they were trying to adapt to having been sexually abused. Since the group members and the therapist were alcoholics, Margaret began to identify with others.

In addition, she was clinically depressed and required three months in residence before the therapeutic blood level of an antidepressant to which she responded was attained. Improvement in outlook and the accomplishment of three months of abstinence from alcohol, along with group bonding, increased Margaret's interest in her own welfare. She consented to live in an AA-oriented halfway house for six months, where she would have additional group and individual counseling as well as vocational rehabilitation.

Marital Sexual Adjustment in Actively Drinking Female Alcoholics

Reciprocal Behavior Pattern in Spouse

Most treatment centers that provide family therapy for alcoholics base this treatment on the principles of Al-Anon. This organization shares the same format and philosophy as AA. It is believed that the spouse has a set of defenses that are the mirror image of those of his alcoholic wife's. The wife unconsciously denies the truth of her alcoholism and so does her husband, who rationalizes her behavior, just as she does. In order to protect the family, the husband "enables" the wife to drink by making excuses for her social or occupational unreliability rather than letting her experience the consequences of her behavior.

Although the syndrome of reciprocal defenses and enabling does occur, and has been witnessed by many clinicians specializing in substance abuse, it has not been verified in refereed journals. Corrigan (1980) and Dahlgren (1979) concluded that husbands may help to maintain their wives' problem drinking by drinking with them. There is some evidence that assortive mating is occurring. Jacob and Bremer (1986) have indicated that alcoholics are more likely to marry other alcoholics than would be expected by chance and that this is as true for male as for female alcoholics. It had previously been supposed that assortive mating among male alcoholics is not found.

Long-Term Outcome in Marriages of Female versus Male Alcoholics

Most studies report a higher rate of divorce among female than male alcoholics (Williams and Klerman 1984; Rimmer 1974).

Dahlgren (1979) reported that the women in a sample comparing 51 marriages in which the wife was alcoholic to a group of alcoholic men were more often widowed than divorced. These marriages were followed over 6 to 12 years. The alcoholics' husbands tended to be older, which might explain the higher rate of widowhood.

Sexual therapy can succeed. It has a tendency to fail if sobriety is not established because of severe psychopathology, lack of commitment to the relationship, or the desire to maintain a drinking status quo on the part of the patients (Powell 1985). With competent sexual therapists and motivated patients, the greatest impediment is the therapists' inability to deal with alcoholism.

Influence of Abstinence from Alcohol on Marriages in which the Female Spouse is Recovering from Alcoholism

Women entering treatment encounter opposition from the family significantly more often than men. Beckman and Amaro (1986) conducted personal interviews with 67 women and 54 men just beginning treatment in a rehabilitation facility. Women received more support from children and parents, whereas men were more often urged by their spouses to seek help. For men, opposition to treatment by their wives "was almost unheard of." This was not the case with women.

Case Histories

Case history 1. Jenny said her husband would refuse to participate in any aspect of her treatment because alcohol was her problem, not his. This proved true. Letters and phone calls from her referring psychiatrist, her attending psychiatrist, and her counselor produced no change in her husband's decision. She reported that, during visiting hours, he had indicated that the drinking problem should be resolved completely by the time she left the hospital. On her first evening after being discharged, her husband asked her whether she wanted wine or beer with dinner.

Case history 2. Mary's husband, John, wanted to be helpful. He insisted on taking his wife on a cruise as soon as her inpatient rehabilitation was completed. Her counselor pointed out that this would delay her entry into the AA community at home and that for six months to a year she would need daily support from AA members. John and Mary had agreed not to tell any of her friends about her alcoholism, and they didn't want to change their plans, which involved another couple. John said that Mary would be safe with him and didn't need anyone else for support. Mary went on the cruise, and felt an extreme craving for alcohol. She entered a hospital-based after-care group and attended AA sporadically, despite group members' urging. She said that her husband resented time away from him at evening meetings and that she might be seen by someone she knew who would gossip about her AA membership. After skipping a few sessions, Mary returned to the group and said that she had been intoxicated at two social gatherings and had begun drinking alone during the day. She refused further treatment.

In spite of willingness to help his spouse continue in her recovery process, a husband must contend with significant changes in routine. AA meetings must not be interfered with. Social engagements involving drinking need to be curtailed. In addition, the couple must interact on a new basis. Many patients have said that they cannot remember talking to their husbands without being under the influence of alcohol. They also do not recall what it is like to engage in sexual activity while sober. In many cases, sexual activity had been curtailed for many years because the patient had been passed out most nights, or had been rendered unattractive as the result of alcohol intoxication. Months often elapse before communication on other levels has been established sufficiently for feelings of affection and sexual attraction to emerge.

When the husband is involved in Al-Anon in conjunction with his wife's attendance at AA, renewal of bonding and mutual understanding come about much more easily. Moreover, socialization with other couples who are members of these groups helps to compensate for the social curtailment necessitated by the wife's effort to remain abstinent from alcohol. However, most husbands resist attending support groups because they think that the need for support is a reflection on their ability to be strong, masculine, and independent. New strategies need development in order to increase the drawing power of Al-Anon for husbands.

Case History

Nancy was exasperated with her husband's constant focus on her drinking. She said that most of their conflict had to do with Bob's self-satisfied, pompous attitude which had driven her to drink. During inpatient treatment she realized that her alcoholism had predated her marriage, which was only of five years' duration. She reflected that she had married Bob because of his sense of humor. His scolding attitude had come about as her drinking became more problematic. Arguments erupted when Bob got home from work. By this time, Nancy had consumed a pint of vodka. Anger distanced them sexually. It was difficult to restore the relationship that had resulted in marriage. Bob and Nancy had marital therapy sessions while Nancy was in the hospital. Nancy was also given a few hours off the hospital grounds with Bob during her last weekend in rehabilitation. They both acknowledged that they got along quite well when alcohol was not involved. Bob had wounded feelings as a result of years of verbal abuse. He had been advised to try some Al-Anon meetings and developed an alliance with another husband in one of his local groups. Nancy had developed positive identification with women in the rehabilitation program and in the AA meetings she had been attending. After Nancy was discharged, she and Bob often attended AA and Al-Anon meetings held at the same times and locations. They reported that their sexual life together took about six months to redevelop. It was now more pleasurable than ever, because of deepening affection and sense of commitment. In addition, Nancy experienced intensified arousal and orgasmic response since she had stopped drinking.

Actively alcoholic husbands are an additional and very severe problem facing married alcoholic women when they leave inpatient treatment. Unless the husbands are abstinent from alcohol and involved in AA themselves, they sabotage the efforts of their wives to stay sober.

Case History

Dan resented his wife's wish to stay sober. She begged him to lock up the alcohol in the house and not to drink in front of her. She knew that looking at the bottles would make it hard for her to resist her intense craving for alcohol. Dan refused to do this because he did not think he should be penalized for his wife's problem. Dan had been arrested twice for driving while intoxicated and had been passed over for a new position at work because of alcohol-related deterioration in his job performance. He often made scenes about feeling neglected before his wife left for AA meetings. After she joined Al-Anon as well as AA, Dan's wife learned to understand that Dan's resistance to her recovery from alcoholism was the result of his need for a drinking companion in order to justify his own urge to drink. She managed not to succumb to drinking. When Dan's company demanded that he either enter a substance abuse rehabilitation facility or lose his job, he was confronted by his own illness. This gave the marriage and the couple's sobriety a chance of survival.

Influence of Chronic Alcoholism on Lesbian Relationships

Lesbian couples share many of the same problems faced by heterosexual couples when one of the partners is alcoholic. The alcoholic lover is quarrelsome, verbally abusive, unreliable, and diminishingly attractive due to the progression of alcoholism. Social engagements may end in an embarrassing scene because the alcoholic partner is drunk.

Finnegan and Cook (1984) describe internalized homophobia among many lesbians, which the authors ascribe to sociohistorical roots as well as to the heterosexually oriented and somewhat homophobic values that the lesbian patients absorbed in their own upbringing. This increases the lowered self-esteem brought about as the result of alcoholism. Since both homosexual partners are highly sensitive to any hint of repulsion because of their sexual preference, therapists must think through their own attitudes and behavior. Therapy for the partners should focus on issues pertaining to alcoholism. Problems with sexual interaction between the partners should await a trial period to establish sobriety. If sexual dysfunction continues to be a source of distress after about six months, the couple should be referred for sexual therapy.

Case History

Tammy had taxed Fran's endurance to the limit. Their house was always a mess because Tammy never picked up her clothes or washed a dish. Fran tried valiantly to keep things in order but it was becoming increasingly impossible. Tammy was now taking at least a sick day a week and Fran had become tired of phoning Tammy's boss to make excuses for her. Friends didn't invite them to parties because Tammy always got drunk and fought with someone. Furthermore, Tammy, who had been fastidious about her appearance when they met six years before, had become bloated and unkempt. She often reeked of alcohol and went several days without a bath. They had made love several times a week in their first two years together but this gradually became less frequent because Tammy got so belligerent when she was drinking. In the past year, sex was nonexistent. Fran was not interested in anyone else. She finally threatened Tammy with termination of their relationship if she didn't stop drinking. They researched rehabilitation centers together as their first joint effort in a long time.

Tammy asked for a female therapist and a female counselor. She was apprehensive about letting anyone know that she was gay but found that her fellow patients and her therapists received the information in a matter-of-fact way. Therapy was based on alcoholism issues. In group therapy, members discussed the way in which alcohol affected all long-term sexual relationships regardless of sexual persuasion. Tammy and Fran were seen together by Tammy's psychiatrist and her substance-abuse counselor. Fran explained her anger and sense of rejection over the years because Tammy appeared more interested in alcohol than in their relationship. She also let Tammy know that her rages and her sloppiness had decreased her interest in Tammy sexually. Tammy was shocked and hurt at first, but integrated this information through individual counseling. She began to pay attention to her appearance. Because she wan't drinking, she lost ten pounds within a month's time. Fran was treated like a spouse and therefore attended group sessions for family members.

She became convinced that alcohol was largely responsible for Tammy's behavior. She also realized that Tammy had probably inherited alcoholism. Her mother had been alcoholic and her grandmother had brought her up. Tammy had not chosen alcohol instead of Fran. She could not have stopped drinking without professional help because her illness had progressed to the point of physical dependence. Fran told Tammy that she was willing to try again but would leave if Tammy drank. Tammy developed a close alliance with Gay AA. As her disposition and sense of responsibility for household tasks improved, she and Fran were able to recapture the friendship that had initially bonded them. They were able to enjoy non-drinking social activities with old friends, such as attending the theatre. Tammy did not think that she could attend a restaurant comfortably for about a year. Gradually, Tammy could withstand seeing others drink without wanting to drink herself. As Tammy and Fran reestablished a pattern of shared pleasant activities, their sexual relationship resumed.

Sexual Adjustment of Single Recovering Female Alcoholics

Heterosexual

If married, nonworking women face stigma and lack of understanding regarding alcoholism, the problems increase in complexity for single women. Analysis of the referral patterns in four different companies revealed that the rate at which female problem drinkers are referred to employee assistance programs by work supervisors is a function of their attitudes toward women and drinking. Men are referred if the supervisor has had positive experience with assistance programs in the past and has noted deterioration of job performance or obvious problems with drinking in the male employee. Supervisors who referred women were "likely to hold stigmatized views of women who drink" (Young, Reichman, and Levy 1987). Female alcoholics legally entitled to receive care from the state are instead jailed in Massachusetts because there is no state alcoholism treatment facility for women (*New York Times*, February 1, 1987).

Single women must begin their non-drinking existence alone. Unless, of course, they live with somebody, they must go home from work to empty rooms. Any new socialization with males has to be done without drinking. Embarking on a serious relationship early in recovery would require concentration, which could distract from the effort to remain sober. Rejection is a frequent trigger for relapse. This leaves single women with limited sexual outlet in their first year of abstinence from alcohol. Finding a partner in AA has been tried often, but the danger is that one of the partners can relapse, which threatens the sobriety of the other. Many women had sexual experiences while drinking which were demeaning and about which they feel ashamed. The therapeutic implication is that they must accept this previous behavior as a symptom of active alcoholism and go on from there. Learning to be sexual in the context of a loving relationship with a caring partner is very difficult for women who have had inhibitions about achieving true intimacy. This is especially true if they have been sexually abused. Therapy should provide a forum for ventilation of anxieties about sex and fostering of self-esteem. This should occur early in treatment because delay leaves hidden and unanswered questions which can lead to drinking for relief. Treatment of specific dysfunctions such as anorgasmia or desire phase disorders should be delayed for six to eight months until physical and perhaps "emotional toxicity" has subsided (Apter-Marsh 1984).

Case History

Melissa was the vice-president of sales for the Northeast in a medium-sized company. Her decision-making had been poor during the six months preceding admission and she was arriving at work progressively later. When traveling for the firm, she managed to be delayed getting back and missed appointments with important clients at her destination. Her boss attributed this to Melissa's distress about vague family pressures. It was only when Melissa noted that she had completely forgotten an important sales agreement that she became frightened enough about her drinking to seek help. She told her boss that, from what she had read about alcoholism, this suggested an alcoholic blackout to her. He was shocked, but consented to let her use the company health plan for inpatient substance-abuse rehabilitation.

Melissa had failed to appear at meetings out of town because she was drunk. Furthermore, she occasionally had been engaged in one-night stands with men who picked her up in hotel bars. She frequently didn't remember what had led up to finding herself in bed with a man she didn't recognize. This had propelled her to research alcoholic blackouts. She knew intellectually that she was drinking too much, but the blackouts forced her to take action. In talking with her therapist, Melissa described her revulsion toward and condemned her own sexual behavior.

Some patients in a weekly women's discussion group had also engaged in sex with partners whom they never would have chosen had they not been drinking. Melissa felt less like a pariah when she could attribute her promiscuity to alcoholism but still doubted that she would be capable of emotional intimacy in a long-term relationship. She noted that her sexual desire was almost completely absent now that she was not drinking. After she was discharged and returned to work, she went to AA and remained abstinent from alcohol. It took about a year, but gradually she noticed that she was daydreaming about sex with a man who had attracted her. During her active drinking, she had always distanced herself from any male companion unless his approach was made when she was already drunk. Drinking had been her only true desire at that time. During the early months of sobriety, it was taking every ounce of energy to maintain sobriety and perform well at her job. As she became more secure about her ability to stay sober, she became receptive to relationships. She had to stay away from activities that involved drinking, but accepted tennis or movie invitations. After two years of sobriety, she became engaged to a man whom she had made fully aware of her alcoholism. She knew that there was always the danger of relapse and felt obligated to make this clear, for his sake as well as hers. Not only was it important that their relationship be without secrets but also, if she couldn't tell her prospective husband about alcoholism, then she was in danger of deceiving herself about it. She had learned that self-deception often led right back to drinking, and she wanted to avoid that at all costs.

Homosexual

Alcoholic lesbians are often obsessed with the fear of loneliness if they are without a current lover. It is frequently difficult for them to focus on the issue of their alcoholism because they are so conscious of the obstacles that they will face in establishing patterns of socialization outside of gay bars. If they are comfortable with their sexual preference, Gay AA is often acceptable to them as a very important source of support as well as an opportunity for socialization. Lesbians who are ambivalent about their sexuality and prefer to consider themselves bisexual cannot tolerate the suggestion of attending Gay AA meetings.

Case History

Jackie had just broken up with her lover, Sarah, and began drinking after six weeks of abstinence. She needed detoxification and came to this center after having been treated at many others during the past ten years. Drinking was always precipitated by a crisis in her love life. Counselors had repeatedly advised that she refrain from major changes such as embarking on a new relationship until she was sufficiently recovered from alcoholism. But Jackie had left every treatment center espousing determination to remain sober, followed shortly thereafter by the triumphant announcement to her counselors that she had finally discovered the person that was meant for her. Unfortunately, these announcements were followed in turn by a rehospitalization after the relationship had gone sour. Jackie was so afraid of being alone that finding a mate had become her main focus. In spite of all the evidence, she didn't see the connection between her relapses and her desperate attempts not to remain single. A counselor finally succeeded in pointing out to her that, since she found new friends so quickly, her fears about loneliness were apparently unrealistic. She realized that she could afford to build up a period of sobriety while being more selective about long-term partners. Jackie had been hesitant about attending Gay AA meetings and didn't think that she could tell her heterosexual sponsor that she was gay. Therefore she had been unable to tell her sponsor about her main relapse trigger of romantic entanglements. A speaker at one of her meetings identified himself as a homosexual and Jackie asked him to be her sponsor. He was able to spot signs of potential trouble for Jackie, and, since he shared the stigma of being homosexual, he also had credibility. So far, Jackie has avoided relapse for a year.

SUMMARY

Since there are important differences between alcohol's effect on the sexuality of female as compared with male alcoholics, the two groups have been allotted separate chapters.

The prevalence of alcoholism in women is either increasing or has been underreported in the past. At Silver Hill Foundation, in terms of total number of admissions for alcoholism per year, half are women. The antecedents of alcoholism in women are thought to be due to affective disorder (Hesselbrock, Meyer, and Keener 1985), role conflict, sexual trauma in childhood, or parental rejection, and seldom merely to genetic vulnerability to alcoholism, as has been postulated in the case of male alcoholics (Cloninger, Bohman, and Sigvardsson 1981; Cadoret, Troughton, and O'Gorman 1987; Goodwin 1985). However, there is some evidence for genetic susceptibility to alcoholism in women (Bohman, Sigvardsson, and Cloninger 1981).

Until recently, women who drank too much were thought to do so in order to experience otherwise absent sexual desire. Sexual dysfunction preceding alcoholism has been ascribed to women alcoholics as the rule rather than the exception. Earlier investigators had considered this to be true of male alcoholics as well (see Chapter 2). There has been a good deal of research evidence refuting the notion that male alcoholics are all latent homosexuals, a commonly held theory until the mid 1970s. Perhaps future studies of women will discern between those who have had antecedent trauma affecting their sexual adaptation and those who are temporarily less interested in sex because they are struggling in their efforts to become sober, as suggested by Apter-Marsh (1984).

Hormonal studies clearly show an adverse influence of alcohol on male sexuality. In women, although alcohol does produce hormonal changes involved in Fetal Alcohol Syndrome, changes resulting in sexual dysfunction such as anorgasmia are not as apparent.

The problems that prevent women from seeking treatment and the barriers to recovery when they do seek help sharply distinguish female from male alcoholics. These problems and barriers largely have to do with the stigma attached to being alcoholic and female. Societal attitudes about women drinkers affect the degree to which spouses, lovers, and employers are willing to accept the need for treatment and aid recovery. While male alcoholics often do encounter stigma about being alcoholic in the workplace, employee assistance programs often help them to overcome this obstacle. Women are less frequently helped by such programs. Women leave their alcoholic husbands far less often than husbands leave their alcoholic wives.

Many of these husbands are alcoholic themselves (Jacob and Bremer 1986).

Because of loneliness, single male and female alcoholics suffer similar adjustment problems. Rejection by potential sexual partners has been reported as a frequent trigger for relapse, and long periods of sexual abstinence while establishing sobriety are often advised as an alternative to this danger. On the other hand, continued isolation is also likely to induce a craving for alcohol. Nobody has developed a definitive solution to this problem. It is advisable to intensify the support from AA and individual counseling for single people as they face this hurdle.

Lesbians and male homosexual alcoholics also share problems in establishing support. Gay AA is helpful for those who are unambivalent about their sexual affiliation. Patients who are in conflict about their sexual identity need to sort out treatment priorities. Concentration on giving up alcohol needs to come first, so that long-term psychotherapy can be meaningful. No amount of therapy has an impact if the patient is preoccupied with obtaining a drink or is hungover, which is why attempts at resolving sexual conflict while actively alcoholic are unproductive.

REFERENCES

Abel, E. L. 1985. *Psychoactive Drugs and Sex* (New York: Plenum Press), pp. 35-48.

Amir, M. 1967. "Alcohol and Forcible Rape." *Br. J. Addict.* 62:219-32.

Apter-Marsh, M. 1984. "The Sexual Behavior of Alcoholic Women While Drinking and During Sobriety." In *Alcoholism and Sexual Dysfunction—Issues in Clinical Management*, edited by D. J. Powell (New York: The Haworth Press), pp. 35-48.

Beckman, L. J., and H. Amaro. 1986. "Personal and Social Difficulties Faced by Women and Men Entering Alcoholism Treatment." *J. Stud. Alcoholism* 47, no. 2:135-45.

Benward, J., and J. Denson-Gerber. 1975. "Incest as a Causative Factor in Anti-Social Behavior: An Exploratory Study." Paper presented at the meeting of the American Academy of Forensic Science, Chicago.

Blume, S. 1986. "Women and Alcohol: A Review." *JAMA* 256, no. 11: 1467-70.

Bohman, M., S. Sigvardsson, and R. Cloninger. 1981. "Maternal Inheritance of Alcohol Abuse: Cross-Fostering Analysis of Adopted Women." *Arch. Gen. Psychiatr.* 38, no. 9:965-69.

Browne-Mayers, A. N., E. E. Seelye, and L. Sillman. 1976. "Psychosocial Study of Hospitalized Middle-Class Alcoholic Women." *Annals N. Y. Acad. Sci.* 273:593-604.

Cadoret, R. J., E. Troughton, and T. W. O'Gorman. 1987. "Genetics and Environmental Factors in Alcohol Abuse and Antisocial Personality." *J. Stud. Alcohol* 48, no. 1:1-8.

Cloninger, C. R., M. Bohman, and S. Sigvardsson. 1981. "Inheritance of Alcohol Abuse: A Cross-Fostering Analysis of Adopted Men." *Arch. Gen. Psychiatr.* 38, no. 8:861-68.

Cohen, F. S., and J. Denson-Gerber. 1982. "A Study of the Relationship Between Child Abuse and Drug Addiction in 178 Patients: Preliminary Results." *Child Abuse Neglect* 6:383-87.

Corrigan, E. M. 1980. *Alcoholic Women in Treatment* (New York: Oxford University Press).

Covington, S. 1986. "Physical, Emotional and Sexual Abuse: Facing the Clinical Challenges of Women Alcoholics." *Focus on Family* (May-June):10-12, 37-44.

Curran, F. 1937. "Personality Studies of Alcoholic Women." *J. Nerv. Ment. Dis.* 86, no. 6:645-67.

Dahlgren, L. 1979. "Female Alcoholics. IV: Marital Situation and Husbands." *Acta Psychiatr. Scand.* 59:59-69.

Filmore, K. M. 1985. "Social Victims of Drinking." *Br. J. Addict.* 80: 307-14.

Finklehor, D. 1980. "Sex Among Siblings: A Survey on Prevalence, Variety, and Effects." *Arch. Sex. Behav.* 9, no. 3:171-94.

Finnegan, D. G., and D. Cook. 1984. "Special Issues Affecting the Treatment of Male Homosexuals and Lesbians." In *Alcoholism & Sexual Dysfunction*, edited by D. J. Pernell (New York: The Haworth Press), pp. 85-94.

Forrest, G. 1983. *Alcoholism and Human Sexuality* (Springfield, IL: Charles C Thomas).

Gallant, D. M. 1986. "A Study of the Victims of Alcohol Abusers." *Alcoholism: Clin. Exptl. Res.* 10, no. 3:358-59.

Gavaler, J. S. 1985. "Effects of Alcohol on Endocrine Function in Postmenopausal Women: A Review." *J. Stud. Alcohol* 40, no. 6:495-516.

Gelinas, D. J. 1983. "The Persisting Negative Effects of Incest." *Psychiatry* 46:312-32.

Goodwin, D. 1985. "Alcoholism and Genetics . . . the Sins of the Fathers." *Arch. Gen. Psychiatr.* 42:171-74.

Heath, D. B. 1986. "Women and Alcohol: Does Gender Make a Difference?" *The Addiction Letter* (December):5-7.

Henderson, J. 1983. "Is Incest Harmful?" *Can. J. Psychiatr.* 28:34-40.

Herman, J., D. Russell, and K. Trocki. 1986. "Long-Term Effects of Incestuous Abuse in Childhood." *Am. J. Psychiatr.* 143, no. 10:1293-96.

Hesselbrock, M. N., R. E. Meyer, and J. G. Keener. 1985. "Psychopathology in Hospitalized Alcoholics." *Arch. Gen. Psychiatr.* 42:1050-55.

Hill, S. Y. 1984. "Vulnerability to the Biomedical Consequences of Alcoholism and Alcohol-Related Problems Among Women." In *Alcohol Problems in Women*, edited by Wilsnak and Beckman (New York: The Guilford Press).

Hugues, J. N., G. Perret, G. Adessi, T. Cosie, and E. Modigliani. 1978. "Effects of Chronic Alcoholism on the Pituitary-Gonadal Function of Women During Menopausal Transition and the Postmenopausal Period." *Biomed. Express* 29:279-83.

Jacob, T., and D. A. Bremer. 1986. "Assortive Mating Among Men and Women Alcoholics." *J. Stud. Alcohol* 47, no. 3:219-22.

Johnson, S. D., L. Gibson, and R. Linden. 1978. "Alcohol and Rape in Winnipeg, 1966-1975." *J. Stud. Alcohol* 39:1887-94.

Kinsey, A., W. Pomeroy, C. Martin, and P. Gebhard. 1953. *Sexual Behavior in the Human Female* (Philadelphia: Saunders).

Lender, M. 1985. "A Special Stigma: Women and Alcoholism in the Late 19th and Early 20th Centuries." In *Alcohol Interventions: Historical and Sociocultural Approaches*, edited by Strug, Piryadarsima, and Heyman (New York, London: The Haworth Press).

Lolli, G. 1961. "Alcohol and the American Woman." In *Social Drinking: The Effects of Alcohol*, edited by G. Lolli (New York: Collier Books).

Malatesta, V. J., R. H. Pollack, T. D. Crotty, and L. J. Peacock. 1982. "Acute Alcohol Intoxication and Female Orgasmic Response." *J. Sex Res.* 18:1-17.

Mandel, L., and S. North. 1982. "Sex Roles, Sexuality and the Recovering Woman Alcoholic: Program Issues." *J. Psychoact. Drugs* 14 (January-June).

Mendelson, J. H. 1986. "Alcohol Effects on Reproductive Function in Women." *Psychiatr. Lett.* 4, no. 7:35-38.

Mendelson, J. H., N. K. Mello, and J. Ellingboe. 1981. "Acute Alcohol Intake and Pituitary-Gonadal Hormones in Normal Human Females." *J. Pharmacol. Exptl. Therapeut.* 218:23-26.

Murphy, W. D., E. Coleman, E. Hoon, and C. Scott. 1980. "Sexual Dysfunction and Treatment of Alcoholic Women." *Sex. Disabil.* 3, no. 4:240-55.

Orme, T. C., and J. Rimmer. 1981. "Alcoholism and Child Abuse: A Review." *J. Stud. Alcohol* 42, no. 3:273-82.

Pinhas, V. 1980. "Sex Guilt and Sexual Control in Women Alcoholics in Early Sobriety." *Sex. Disabil.* 3, no. 4:256-72.

Powell, D. J. 1985. "Management of Sexual Dysfunction." In *Practical Approaches to Alcoholism Psychotherapy*, edited by Zimberg, Wallace, and Blume (New York: Plenum Press).

Rimmer, J. 1974. "Psychiatric Illness in Husbands of Alcoholics." *Q. J. Stud. Alcohol* 35:281-83.

Rohsenow, D., R. Corbet, and D. Devine. 1986. "Molested as Children: The Hidden Contribution to Alcohol and Substance Abuse." Presented at the annual meeting of the American Medical Society on Alcoholism and Other Drug Dependencies, San Francisco.

Rose, D. S. 1986. " 'Worse than Death': Psychodynamics of Rape Victims and the Need for Psychotherapy." *Am. J. Psychiatr.* 143, no. 7:817-24.

Sandmaier, M. 1980. *The Invisible Alcoholic: Women and Alcohol Abuse in America* (New York: McGraw-Hill).

Underhill, B. L. 1986. "Issues Relevant to After-Care Programs for Women." *Alcohol, Health Res. World* (Fall):46-47, 73.

Van Thiel, D., J. Gavaler, and R. Lester. 1977. "Ethanol: A Gonadal Toxin in the Female." *Drug Alcohol Depend.* 2:363-80.

Williams, C. N., and L. V. Klerman. 1984. "Female Alcohol Abuse: Its Effects on the Family." In *Alcohol Problems in Women*, edited by Wilsnak and Beckman (New York: The Guilford Press).

Wilson, G. T., and D. M. Lawson. 1976. "The Effect of Alcohol on Sexual Arousal in Women." *J. Abnorm. Psychol.* 85, no. 3:489-97.

______. 1978. "Expectancies, Alcohol and Sexual Arousal in Women." *J. Abnorm. Psychol.* 87, no. 3:358-67.

Young, D. W., W. R. Reichman, and M. F. Levy. 1987. "Differential Referral of Women and Men to Employee Assistance Programs: The Role of Supervisory Attitudes." *J. Stud. Alcohol* 48, no. 1:22-28.

5

Influence of Other Substances on Sexual Response

INTRODUCTION

In the past ten years there have been fewer "pure alcoholics" seeking treatment under age 40. Although alcohol remains popular consistently, other drugs are abused along with it. Depending on the current drug fad, the other substances belong in the sedative-hypnotic, opioid, amphetamine and cocaine, or cannabis groups. Often a patient abuses a combination of drugs from three or four different categories, each of which has a different set of effects on sexuality. In the past two years, the most frequent drug problem in addition to alcohol has been cocaine. Because a drug's sexual effect varies according to its impact on the neuroendocrine system characteristic of the pharmacologic group to which it belongs, each drug category will be dealt with separately in this chapter.

SEDATIVE-HYPNOTICS

Alcohol belongs to the group of sedative-hypnotics, as do barbiturates, benzodiazepines, and barbiturate-like substances, such as methaqualone (Quaaludes), chloral hydrate, methprylon (Noludar), ethchlorvynol (Placidyl), glutethemide (Doriden), and meprobamate. There is cross-tolerance and cross-dependence among these drugs.

In the 1970s, Quaaludes were thought to enhance sexual experience, and "luding out" became a familiar phrase for a brief period (Ayer 1972; Inaba et al. 1973). Several survey studies at that time revealed that college students and patients at drug clinics believed methaqualone to be a social/sexual disinhibitor (Gerald and Schwirian

1973; Kochansky et al. 1975). This was especially true of female subjects (Kochansky et al. 1975; Parr 1976; Gay et al. 1982). Although methaqualone was used to enhance sex, subjects reported that its actual effect was similar to that of alcohol (Gay et al. 1982). Studies in animals suggest an increase in arousal, but there is no direct evidence of this effect in human beings (Abel 1985). Recently, methaqualone has decreased in popularity, so that there is no topical impetus for studies of its neuroendocrine impact on sexual functioning.

Case History

Ted was brought to the hospital accompanied by his parents. He had been suspended from college and had suffered a back injury after passing out while driving a car under the influence of Quaaludes. He had just been released from the orthopedic ward of a general hospital, where substance-abuse rehabilitation had been advised. After becoming involved in the treatment program, he revealed that "ludes" were used recreationally among the student body because of their aphrodisiac properties. He had had several falls and one previous car accident as a result of Quaalude overdose and had begun using it daily to the point of physiological dependence. Instead of experiencing aphrodisiac effects of methaqualone, he always took several pills rapidly and passed out at parties where the drug was being offered.

Most reports about benzodiazepines do not mention sexual effects. Abel (1985), in a recent review of the literature, concludes that benzodiazepines probably have no direct effect on human sexuality. However, there are some anecdotal reports suggesting that benzodiazepines depress sexual arousal and function. This hypothesis is arrived at by extrapolating the results of withdrawal from benzodiazepines. Nutt, Hackman, and Hawton (1986) describe two cases, both women, in which increased libido and orgasmic function occurred after benzodiazepine withdrawal. In both cases, sexual function again diminished when the patients were restarted on diazepam and temazepam, respectively. The second patient experienced "almost constant sexual arousal which was only slightly relieved by sexual intercourse" several months after withdrawal.Four months after temazepam was discontinued for the second time, this woman's libido returned to its pre-morbid level. Norepinephrine rebound is postulated as the mechanism for the markedly increased sexual arousal during benzodiazepine withdrawal. Riley and Riley (1986) demonstrated that alprazolam interfered with orgasmic function in one patient.

Barbiturates are not highly rated by drug users in terms of sexual enhancement (Gay and Shepard 1972; Gay et al. 1982). Conclusions about hormonal effects of barbiturates are conflicting. In a double-blind study, Linnoila et al. (1980) did not find a significant alteration in testosterone levels of human males after they were given 100 mg of pentobarbital as compared with placebo. Barbiturates increase testosterone levels in monkeys, and decrease levels in dogs and rats (Abel 1985; Cicero and Badger 1977). In female animals, LH is decreased by a direct effect on the action of LHRH in the hypothalamus. Ovulation is inhibited in rats (Abel 1985).

OPIOIDS

Heroin initially helps men who suffer from premature ejaculation because it delays orgasm. With chronic use, men have absent libido because of decreased testosterone, and impotence as the result of decreased LH (Smith et al. 1982; Abel 1985; Cohen 1981). In the questionnaire and interview study of 500 heroin addicts by Smith et al. (1982), dyspareunia was the primary sexual dysfunction among women, followed by anorgasmia and amenorrhea. After cessation of use, women returned to sexual functioning attained prior to use of heroin.

Mirin et al. (1980), in three sequential studies, concluded that heroin use in men results in an acute suppression of LH with a secondary drop in testosterone. This correlates with the time course of the tension-reducing effects of heroin and suggests that drive reduction is an important component of opiate reenforcement. Their subjects reported that a single dose produces a brief but intense euphoria which has been likened to orgasm. Smith et al. (1982) stated that withdrawal from heroin led to rebound hypersexuality with spontaneous erections and frequent "wet dreams."

Crowley and Simpson (1978) noted that methadone decreased testosterone, FSH, and LH, as well as seminal vesicle and prostate secretion in males. Effects of methadone were less clear among the women in their population (31 men and 17 women). The women reported regularized menses as compared with their condition while on heroin. Improvement in menstrual regularity with methadone as compared with heroin had been noted in earlier studies. Blatman (1973) suggested that better nutritional status among methadone users could account for this phenomenon. Hanbury, Cohen, and Stimmel (1977), in a questionnaire study of 50 male narcotic addicts treated with methadone, found that 33 percent reported sexual dysfunction. Inadequate sexual functioning with heroin use had been reported by 12 of the 17 men who experienced dysfunction while on methadone. Failure to achieve orgasm was the most frequent complaint, followed by erectile failure and diminished libido. These side effects were independent of methadone dosage. Similar hormonal depression of testosterone and LH with associated sexual dysfunction has been reported with codeine, propoxyphene, and oxycodone (Smith et al. 1982).

Naltrexone, a narcotic antagonist, produced recurrent spontaneous erections in three of eight men with no prior history of narcotic use (Mendelson et al. 1979). This effect did not occur when placebo was administered. Abbot et al. (1984) demonstrated that naltrexone increased LH in noncastrated as opposed to castrated male rhesus monkeys. Increase of LH in monkeys receiving naloxone, a quicker-acting antagonist, was insignificant. An increase in testosterone always accompanied increases in LH.

FSH levels are not affected significantly by opioids (Abel 1985). Prolactin levels are increased by administration of narcotics (Gold et al. 1978; Mendelson et al. 1980) and decreased by narcotic antagonists and narcotic withdrawal (Gold et al. 1978, 1981).

There have been psychoanalytic hypotheses proposed to explain the lack of sexual drive among narcotics addicts, most notably Sandor Rado's theory of "alimentary orgasm," in which the sensation of a full stomach produced by injection of a narcotic substance is substituted for the pleasure induced by sexual activity (Rado 1926) and the needle is symbolic of the penis. No experimental studies have yet substantiated these ideas (Abel 1985).

Endogeonous opioids such as met-enkephalin are said to inhibit dopamine-stimulated release of LHRH from the hypothalamus. Morphine replicates this action. Inhibition of LHRH release via blockage of dopamine is reversed by naloxone, an opiate antagonist (Rotsztejn et al. 1978; Abel 1985). If luteinizing hormone-releasing hormone is unavailable, then pituitary release of luteinizing hormone is affected negatively, which will in turn decrease stimulation of gonads to release testosterone. Thus sexual dysfunction among narcotics users is thought to be the result of direct pharmacologic action on the central nervous system, and not on the gonads.

COCAINE AND AMPHETAMINES

Cocaine

At low doses cocaine produces a rush akin to sexual excitement. It stimulates release of dopamine, bringing about increased pleasure and alertness. With more chronic use, dopamine re-uptake by dopamine neuroreceptors is blocked. Norepinephrine re-uptake by presynaptic terminals is inhibited as well. In addition, serotonin production is decreased. These neurotransmitter depletions bring about dysphoria with associated reduction of libido. New cocaine users may appreciate the advantage of delayed ejaculation and orgasm because sexual activity can be prolonged. Cocaine can produce spontaneous ejaculation without genital stimulation. With chronic use, men have difficulty maintaining an erection and ejaculating (Cregler and Mark 1986; Gold and Dackis 1984; Siegel 1982; Smith, Wesson, and Apter-Marsh 1984).

Transient hypertension accompanying cocaine use causes peripheral vasoconstriction, resulting in impaired blood flow to the fetus during pregnancy which, along with increased norepinephrine levels, can bring about uterine contractions and spontaneous abortion. Recreational use of cocaine during pregnancy exposes infants to higher rates of congenital malformation, perinatal mortality, and neurobehavioral impairment (Cregler and Mark 1986; Chasoff et al. 1985).

Cocaine abusers frequently report disinterest in sex by the time they have been referred for treatment.

Case Histories

Case history 1. Malcolm, a 38-year-old stockbroker, sought substance-abuse rehabilitation after he had been free-basing cocaine for two years and snorting it for five years. In the initial days of cocaine use, he snorted it only on weekends during social gatherings. He enjoyed the "high" and found that it enhanced heterosexual encounters because he could prolong ejaculation, while, at the same time, experiencing heightened sexual awareness. After a year of sporadic use, he went on weekend binges in which he snorted up to one-eighth of an ounce of cocaine in a 48-hour period. Use was almost continuous because he could not bear the dysphoria that occurred when the effect wore off several minutes after snorting. During this time he was engaged in sexual marathons with multiple partners. Gradually, his work suffered because of the severe lethargy and depression he experienced when "crashing" during the days that he didn't use cocaine. He began not showing up at his office until mid-week and functioning responsibly for three days, only to repeat the cycle the following weekend. He became suspicious that his partners were reporting him to the FBI in an effort to divest him of his partnership. This paranoia was especially pronounced while bingeing. He lost 20 pounds. When he began hallucinating sounds of guns fired by the FBI, he was sometimes aware that this was due to cocaine excitability and attempted to calm himself down with as much as 60 mg of Valium per day prescribed for him by well-meaning internists to whom he had complained of nervousness due to job stress.

He was no longer experiencing any sexual pleasure when "high." Erection and ejaculation were virtually impossible and his cocaine craving persisted in spite of acknowledged absence of libido. When his partners finally forced him to seek treatment or resign, he sought admission to the hospital.

Case history 2. Tammy, a 25-year-old cosmetics firm executive, had been to multiple therapists for six years in an effort to stop using cocaine, but was never able to stay drug-free for more than two weeks. After her current drug-dealing boyfriend was arrested and one friend died from cocaine-induced cardiac arrest, she became frightened enough to arrange for inpatient treatment.

She had always been a high achiever and was well regarded at work. However, her first interest in cocaine had stemmed from its success in suppressing her appetite for food. Self-esteem was almost completely predicated on physical appearance, particularly slenderness. Her mother was quoted as saying things like, "You'd be really pretty if you weighed 10 pounds less" or "You look great; you must have lost weight." Her parents never appeared to notice her excellent grades and her career advancement. She thought that her father was totally uninterested in her and completely immersed in his work, so that nothing she did ever pleased either parent.

In high school and college she seemed attracted only to men who took drugs. She had begun drinking beer and smoking marijuana in high school as regular weekend activities. In college she used cocaine if offered to her by a boyfriend and found that orgasm was delayed and seemed more intense and prolonged. She also experienced intense sexual excitement during the 5 to 15 minutes of the drug's effect. By the time she graduated from college, she began living with a man whose entire living was made from drug dealing. He was often physically abusive and forced her to have group sex with both men and women. By this time she was using huge amounts of cocaine nightly and was willing to submit to anything as long as she was given the drug as a reward.

When she entered the hospital, she recounted these drug-related sexual experiences and said that they intensified her sense of worthlessness. After the first few months of daily cocaine use, she had only engaged in sex for maintenance of her drug supply and no longer experienced any sexual desire or pleasure.

Because of progressive sexual dysfunction, consisting of delayed ejaculation and inability to achieve orgasm among users of large quantities of cocaine, exotic sexual practices are resorted to in the hope that orgasm will become possible with the additional stimulation of deviant behavior. Two male patients told this author that, under the influence of cocaine, they often masturbated while attired in lace underwear. They were horrified at their own behavior and had never cross-dressed prior to cocaine use.

Amphetamines

Low doses are said to produce increased libido and delayed ejaculation with prolonged erection. Women have reported heightened sexual desire and prolonged pelvic thrusting at low dose levels (Smith, Buxton, and Dammon 1978). At higher doses, men and women may have difficulty achieving orgasm. The intravenous route can induce a "pharmacogenic orgasm" which some users have substituted for sex. Behavior that is considered deviant, as compared with what the amphetamine user had done before, also occurs. This consists of group sex, marathon sex, or the choice of a same-sex partner. With chronic use at high doses men develop impotence and women become anorgasmic (Abel 1985). Amphetamines have not been used as extensively as cocaine in recent years. Methylene Dioxy Methyl Amphetamine

(MDMA) has emerged on the streets as a new aphrodisiac, although it simply consists of a methyl group added to a side-chain of MDA (3,4-methylene-dioxy-amphetamine), which is an old drug. It has psychedelic properties similar to those of LSD, and despite anecdotal claims about its ability to produce feelings of love for one's sexual partner, it is hard to understand why it is any more of a love potion than other amphetamines of similar molecular structure (Cohen, 1985b). In high doses, amphetamines produce schizophrenic-like symptoms because they mimic norepinephrine and dopamine. In this respect MDMA is also not unlike other amphetamines. Cocaine and amphetamines differ only in their duration of action. Cocaine wears off in 5 to 15 minutes in contrast to amphetamines, which are long-acting. Like the amphetamines, cocaine inhibits re-uptake of norepinephrine into presynaptic terminals. Effects on sexual functioning produced by amphetamines and cocaine are almost identical.

MARIJUANA

For centuries, marijuana has been associated with sexual activity, but there have been few laboratory studies to substantiate the positive and negative effects on sexuality claimed on the basis of anecdotal evidence (Abel 1985).

There have been some reports of decreased testosterone in males who have smoked marijuana. Kolodny et al. (1974) reported a decrease in plasma testosterone after chronic and heavy use. Later studies, which have measured secretion of LH and FSH as well as testosterone, have been inconclusive (Ehrenkranz and Hembree 1986; Hembree et al. 1979; Mendelson and Mello 1984). In rats there is a consistent lowering of testosterone levels after exposure to cannibis (Abel 1985). Kolodny et al. (1974) reported an increase in testosterone levels in human male marijuana users who were given human chorionic gonadotropin (hCG). This suggests that Leydig cell functioning is intact. Daltiero, Bartke, and Burstein (1977) incubated rat testes with delta-9 THC and hCG and noted decreased testosterone secretion. These disparate results have yet to be explained (Abel 1985). There are some reports of decrease in sperm motility and changes in sperm morphology accompanying marijuana use (Dalterio et al. 1982). However, later studies revealed conflicting results, ranging from marked change to no change in reproductive capacity (Ehrenkranz and Hembree 1986; Abel 1985). Two studies indicate increased incidence of gynecomastia in male marijuana smokers, with associated increase in prolactin secretion (Ehrenkranz and Hembree 1986). Studies in human males on research wards are confounded by the inability of the investigators to control sexual behavior when the subjects were not under direct scrutiny. Intercourse with female visitors and masturbation could deplete the sperm count, unbeknownst to the researchers. Animal studies often fail to take nutritional status of the rat subjects into account (Abel 1985).

Studies of the hormonal effects of marijuana smoking in women have been infrequent and inconclusive. Recent studies suggest that cannabis may produce fetal malformations (Cohen 1986). In female monkeys, there is an apparent tolerance that develops to the disruptive effects of cannabis on the primate menstrual cycle (C. G. Smith et al. 1983).

Most of the experimental data concern hormonal regulation and reproductive functioning in marijuana users. Information about the effects of cannabis on human sexual behavior are derived through questionnaires, with no laboratory behavioral studies to corroborate them as yet (Gay et al. 1977; Goode 1972).

SUMMARY

In general, drugs in all categories do not earn their reputation as aphrodisiacs. Sedative-hypnotics have CNS effects similar to alcohol. In low doses, relaxation and euphoria decrease shyness and bring about heightened sexual pleasure, which may be the result of expectation rather than a true pharmacologic effect. Certain sedative-hypnotics, particularly methaqualone, have been designated as sexual disinhibitors, and "luding out" was popular among college students for a short time in the late 1970s. There are some reports suggesting increased arousal in animals, but not in humans. Except for some recent case reports, describing rebound sexuality after withdrawal from benzodiazepines (which suggests that benzodiazepines resemble alcohol in depressing sexual function), most investigators have concluded that this group of drugs has minimal sexual effects. Reports about the neuroendocrine effects of barbiturates vary with the animal being studied.

Opioids delay orgasm, and bring about decreased libido and impotence as a result of depressed LH and testosterone. Rebound libido often occurs during opioid withdrawal. The effects on women are less clear. Heroin is thought to disrupt menstrual cycles, but for reasons that are still unexplained, methadone sometimes regularizes menses.

Cocaine in low doses, in the initial stages of an individual's cocaine use, actually intensifies desire through noradrenergic and dopaminergic neuronal firing with blockage of neuroreceptor re-uptake. In later stages, these neurotransmitters are depleted, resulting in anorgasmia, impotence, and libido depression. Amphetamines are longer-acting but have essentially the same effect.

Marijuana was once highly touted as an aphrodisiac. Reports of its actual influence on human sexuality are conflicting and inconclusive.

REFERENCES

Abbot, D., S. D. Holmar, M. Berman, D. Neff, and R. Gay. 1984. "Effects of Opiate Antagonists on Hormones and Behavior of Male and Female Rhesus Monkeys." *Arch. Sex. Behav.* 13, no. 1:1-25.

Abel, E. L. 1985. *Psychoactive Drugs and Sex* (New York: Plenum Press).

Ayer, S. 1972. "Luding Out." *N. Engl. J. Med.* 287:51.

Blatman, S. 1973. "Methadone Effects on Pregnancy and the Newborn." Proceedings of the Third National Conference on Methadone Treatment, pp. 842-45.

Blum, K. 1984. "Influence of Psychopharmacologic Agents on Sexual Function: 'Psychopharmacology.' " In *Handbook of Abusable Drugs* (New York: Gardner Press), Chapter 20, pp. 645-61.

Chasoff, I. J., W. J. Burns, S. H. Scholl, and K. A. Burns. 1985. "Cocaine Use in Pregnancy." *N. Engl. J. Med.* 313:666-9.

Cicero, T. J., and T. M. Badger. 1977. "A Comparative Analysis of the Effects of Narcotics, Alcohol, and the Barbiturates on the Hypothalamic-Pituitary-Gonadal Axis." *Adv. Exptl. Med. Biol.* 85B: 94-115.

Cohen, S. 1981. *Substance Abuse Problems* (New York: Haworth Press).

______. 1985a. "Marijuana and Reproductive Function." *Drug Abuse and Alcoholism Newsletter* (Vista Hill Foundation) 13, no. 10.

______. 1985b. "They Call It Ecstacy." *Drug Abuse and Alcoholism Newsletter* (Vista Hill Foundation) 14, no. 6.

______. 1986. "Marijuana Research: Selected Recent Findings." *Drug Abuse and Alcoholism Newsletter* (Vista Hill Foundation) 15, no. 1.

Cregler, L. J., and H. Mark. 1986. "Medical Complications of Cocaine Abuse." *N. Engl. J. Med.* 315, no. 23:1495-1500.

Crowley, T. J., and R. Simpson. 1978. "Methadone Dose and Human Sexual Behavior." *Internat. J. Addict.* 13, no. 2:285-95.

Dalterio, S., F. Badr, A. Bartke, and D. Mayfield. 1982. "Cannabinoids in Male Mice: Effects on Fertility and Spermatogenesis." *Science* 216:313-16.

Dalterio, S., A. Bartke, and S. Burstein. 1977. "Cannabinoids Inhibit Testosterone Secretion *In Vitro*." *Science* 196:1472.

Ehrenkranz, J. R. L., and W. C. Hembree. 1986. "Effects of Marijuana on Male Reproductive Function." *Psychiatr. Annals* 16, no. 4: 243-48.

Gay, G. R., J. A. Newmeyer, R. A. Elion, and S. Wieder. 1977. "The Sensuous Hippie. Part I: Drug/Sex Practices in Haight-Ashbury." *Drug Forum* 6:27.

Gay, G. R., J. Newmeyer, M. Perry, G. Johnson, and M. Kurland. 1982. "Love and Haight: The Sensuous Hippie Revisited. Drug/Sex Practices in San Francisco, 1980-81." *J. Psychoact. Drugs* 14:11-123.

Gay, G. R., and C. W. Shepard. 1972. "Sex in the Drug Culture." *Med. Aspects Hum. Sex.* 6:28-47.

Gerald, M. C., and P. M. Schwirian. 1973. "Non-Medical Use of Methaqualone." *Arch. Gen. Psychiatr.* 28:627-31.

Gold, M. S., and C. A. Dackis. 1984. "New Insights and Treatments: Opiate Withdrawal and Cocaine Addiction." *Clin. Ther.* 7:6-21.

Gold, M. S., A. L. C. Pottash, I. Extein, and H. D. Kleber. 1981. "Dopamine and Serum Prolactin in Methadone Withdrawal." *NIDA Research no. 34, Problems of Drug Dependence.* Proceedings of the 42nd Annual Scientific Meeting, National Institute of Drug Abuse, pp. 367-72.

Gold, M. S., D. E. Redmond, R. K. Donabedian, F. K. Goodwin, and I. Extein. 1978. "Increase in Serum Prolactin by Exogenous and Endogenous Opiates: Evidence for Antidopamine and Antipsychotic Effects." *Am. J. Psychiatr.* 135:1415-16.

Goode, E. 1972. "Drug Use and Sexual Activity on a College Campus." *Am. J. Psychiatr.* 128:1272.

Hanbury, R., M. Cohen, and B. Stimmel. 1977. "Adequacy of Sexual Performance in Men Maintained on Methadone." *Am. J. Drug Alcohol Abuse* 4, no. 1:13-20.

Hembree, W. C., G. G. Nahas, P. Zeidenberg, and H. F. S. Huang. 1979. "Changes in Human Spermatozoa Associated with High-Dose Marihuana Smoking." In *Marihuana: Biological Effects*, edited by G. G. Nahas and W. Patton (Oxford: Pergamon Press).

Inaba, D. S., G. R. Gay, J. A. Newmayer, and C. Whitehead. 1973. "Methaqualone Abuse: 'Luding Out.' " *JAMA* 224:1505.

Kochansky, G. E., T. S. Hemenway, C. Salzman, and R. I. Shader. 1975. "Methaqualone Abusers: A Preliminary Survey of College Students." *Dis. Nerv. Syst.* 36:348-51.

Kolodny, R., P. Lessin, T. Gelson, W. H. Masters, and S. Cohen. 1976. "Depression of Plasma Testosterone with Acute Marijuana Administration." In *The Pharmacology of Marijuana*, edited by M. C. Braude and S. Szara (New York: Raven Press), pp. 217-25.

Kolodny, R. C., W. H. Masters, R. M. Kolodner, and J. Toro. 1974. "Depression of Plasma Testosterone After Chronic Intensive Marijuana Use." *N. Engl. J. Med.* 290:872-74.

Linnoila, M., P. N. Prinz, C. J. Wonsowicz, and J. Leppaluioto. 1980. "Effect of Moderate Doses of Ethanol and Phenobarbital on Pituitary and Thyroid Hormones and Testosterone." *Br. J. Addict.* 75: 207.

Mendelson, J. H., J. Ellingboe, J. C. Kuehnle, and N. K. Mello. 1979. "Effects of Naltrexone on Mood and Neuroendocrine Function in Normal Adult Males." *Psychoendocrinology* 2:231-36.

Mendelson, J. H., J. Ellingboe, J. C. Kuehnle, and N. K. Mello. 1980. "Heroin and Naltrexone Effects on Pituitary-Gonadal Hormones in Man." *J. Pharmacol. Exptl. Therapeut.* 214:503-6.

Mendelson, J. H., and N. K. Mello. 1984. "Effects of Marijuana on Neuroendocrine Hormones in Human Males and Females." In *Marijuana: Effects on the Endocrine and Reproductive Systems*, edited by M. C. Braude and J. P. Ludford. N.I.D.A. Research monograph no. 44, Rockville, MD.

Mirin, S. M., R. E. Meyer, J. H. Mendelson, and J. Ellingboe. 1980. "Opiate Use and Sexual Function." *Am. J. Psychiatr.* 137, no. 8:909-15.

Nutt, D., A. Hackman, and K. Hawton. 1986. "Increased Sexual Function in Benzodiazepine Withdrawal." *Lancet*, November 8, pp. 1101-2.

Parr, D. 1976. "Sexual Aspects of Drug Abuse in Narcotic Addicts." *Br. J. Addict.* 71:261-68.

Rado, S. 1926. "The Psychic Effects of Intoxicants: An Attempt to Evolve a Psychoanalytic Theory of Morbid Cravings." *Internat. J. Psychoanal.* 7:396-413.

Riley, A. J., and E. J. Riley. 1986. "The Effect of Single Dose Diazepam on Female Sexual Response Induced by Masturbation." *Sex. Marital Ther.* 1:49-53.

Rotsztejn, W. H., S. V. Drouva, E. Pattou, and C. Kordan. 1978. "Effects of Morphine on the Basal and the Dopamine-Induced Release of LHRH from Mediobasal Hypothalamic Fragments *In Vitro*." *J. Pharmacol.* 50:285-86.

Siegel, R. 1982. "Cocaine and Sexual Dysfunction: The Curse of Mama Coca." *J. Psychoact. Drugs* 14:71-74.

Smith, C. G., R. G. Almirez, J. Berenberg, and R. H. Asch. 1983. "Tolerance Develops to the Disruptive Effects of Delta-9-Tetrahydrocannabinol on Primate Menstrual Cycle." *Science* 219:1453-55.

Smith, D. E., M. E. Buxton, and G. Dammon. 1978. "Amphetamine Abuse and Sexual Dysfunction: Clinical and Research Considerations." In *Amphetamine Use, Misuse, and Abuse: Proceedings of the National Amphetamine Conference*, edited by D. E. Smith, D. R. Wesson, M. E. Buxton, R. B. Seymour, J. T. Ungerleider, J. P. Morgan, A. J. Mandell, and G. Jara (Boston, MA: G.K. Hall and Co.), pp. 228-48.

Smith, D. E., C. Moser, D. R. Wesson, M. Apter-Marsh, M. E. Buxton, J. V. Davison, M. Orgel, and J. Buffam. 1982. "A Clinical Guide to the Diagnosis and Treatment of Heroin-Related Sexual Dysfunction." *J. Psychoact. Drugs* 14:91-99.

Smith, D. E., D. R. Wesson, and M. Apter-Marsh. 1984. "Cocaine and Alcohol Sexual Dysfunction in Patients with Addictive Diseases." *J. Psychoact. Drugs* 16:359-61.

Tennes, K. 1984. "Effects of Marijuana on Pregnancy and Fetal Development in the Human." In *Marijuana Effects on the Endocrine and Reproductive Systems*, NIDA Research Monograph no. 44, edited by M. D. Braude and J. P. Ludford (Rockford, MD), pp. 15-24.

Summary

Until very recently, the fields of substance abuse and human sexuality did not overlap. Therapists and researchers engaged in the treatment and study of substance abuse rarely noted that sexual dysfunction was a drug side effect frequently affecting the lives of their patients. Those engaged in the study and treatment of sexual dysfunction paid some, but not enough, attention to the need for obtaining a substance-use history from their patients.

In the last 15 years more careful attention has been paid to collecting data and gathering experimental evidence about the impact of substance use and abuse on human sexual functioning.

Except for one chapter devoted to other frequently abused substances (Chapter 5), this book focuses on the way in which alcohol influences human sexuality.

Although alcohol intoxication produces sexual dysfunction, alcohol is highly regarded as an aphrodisiac. For centuries bacchanalian sexual behavior and impotence have both been attributed to alcohol. In contemporary surveys of drug usage, the population samples often choose alcohol for its alleged property of inducing social disinhibition with facilitation of increased sexual risk-taking. Actual effects of alcohol are dependent on dosage. Behavioral psychological studies measuring alcohol's direct effect on sexual functioning indicate that, at low doses, expectation of enhanced functioning in the presence of alcohol produces increased penile tumescence in men who are responding to laboratory-induced erotic stimuli. Control subjects who receive placebo in the belief that they are drinking alcohol also achieve increased penile tumescence in response to erotic stimuli. With larger doses, decrease in penile tumescence occurs regardless of expectation (Briddell and Wilson 1976; Lansky and Wilson 1981; Wilson 1977, 1981; Wilson and Niaura 1984). This correlates with accompanying hormonal changes. Testosterone and luteinizing hormone are decreased in male alcoholics. Testosterone is decreased after single episodes of drinking in nonalcoholic males as well (Ylikahri et al. 1974). Masters and Johnson (1970) reported that single episodes of heavy drinking with resultant inability to achieve erection or to ejaculate often lead to performance fears, which are, aside from premature ejaculation, the most frequent cause of secondary impotence.

Although alcohol does affect male social drinkers, the changes in sexual functioning as a result of chronic alcoholism are far more severe.

Male alcoholics suffer from increased clearance and depletion of testosterone, increased clearance of estrogen, and decreased luteinizing hormone. Feminization comes about as the result of direct toxic effects of alcohol, not only on the liver but also on the Leydig cells of the testes and the hypothalamic-pituitary-gonadal axis. Lack of sexual desire has been reported by some male alcoholics who have been drinking pathologically for at least 10 years. Some investigators still think that latent homosexuality, which predates the alcoholism, is the cause for this absence of interest in sex. Other investigators have noted normal pre-morbid sexual functioning with decreased libido as the result of diminution or absence of erectile capacity in their alcoholic population samples. To postulate a universal psychodynamic etiology for alcoholism seems outdated in the face of evidence of the hormonal disruption brought about by massive alcohol ingestion over time. In addition, there is evidence that alcoholism is hereditary. Goodwin (1985) reports that sons of alcoholic fathers have a fourfold greater chance of developing alcoholism as compared with controls in adopted-away twin studies. Genetic determinants have also been suggested by Cloninger, Bohman, and Sigvardsson (1981) and by Cadoret, Troughton, and O'Gorman (1987).

Alcoholism affects sexual relationships indirectly as well as directly. Years of living with an emotionally unreliable person can cool sexual desire in the alcoholics' marital partner or lover. Rehabilitation of the alcoholic is more likely to be effective if the spouse or partner is included in the treatment. Education, individual and family therapy, as well as introduction to self-help groups like Al-Anon, Alateen, and Adult Children of Alcoholics helps in fostering recognition of the problem. This facilitates better understanding of the patient, improves the partners' self-esteem through positive identification with others in the same situation, and can lead to renewed bonding with the alcoholic if he or she remains abstinent.

Gradually it is being recognized that women alcoholics comprise a substantial portion of the alcoholic population deserving of focused rehabilitation efforts and research. The numbers of nonalcoholic female social drinkers have increased in the past 40 years. After Fetal Alcohol Syndrome became publicized, attention began to be paid to this group of consumers. Female sexuality in general is less well understood than male sexual response, which is much easier to observe and document. After Masters and Johnson first delineated the steps of female orgasmic response, with ensuing revived debate about clitoral versus vaginal orgasm, a methodology emerged for direct measurement of sexual arousal in females with the development of the vaginal plethysmograph. This made it possible to measure feminine arousal to stimuli under a variety of experimental conditions, including exposure to alcohol. As with males, the factor of social expectation regarding alcohol was taken into account. Unlike male social drinkers, women manifest decreased labial engorgement in response to erotic stimuli if they have been exposed to alcohol regardless of pretesting beliefs about the effects of alcohol on sexuality. They also differ from male social drinkers in their ability to observe the actual effects of alcohol on their sexual responsiveness. Women think that their sexual arousal is facilitated by alcohol even when physiological measurements of labial engorgement run directly opposite to those perceptions. Male subjects are accurate in assessing decrements in their arousability (Wilson and Lawson 1976; Wilson, Lawson and Abrams 1978; Malatesta et al. 1979).

Sexual response in female alcoholics is a subject that is just emerging as a research area. Therefore, certain conclusions that have been reached in studies of male alcoholic populations are still a matter for debate and further investigation in regard to women. For example, the long-term hormonal effects of chronic alcoholism in women are ill-defined. By extrapolation it would appear that alcohol does induce hormonal consequences. It is known that exogenous estrogen administration may cause fetal abnormalities. The role of alcohol in modifying estrogen metabolism in early pregnancy is being investigated as a possible mechanism for the Fetal Alcohol Syndrome.

It has long been assumed that female alcoholics have immature and conflicted gender identity, with lack of interest in sex. Most populations have been studied during active drinking or in early recovery. Apter-Marsh (1984) studied 61 women in several stages of recovery, which included a point at which four years of sobriety had been reached. She concluded that sexual adjustment was a function of the time in the recovery process that a subject was interviewed. In many studies, women had histories of having been raped while drinking or of experiencing incest. Women with these histories had more troubled psychosexual adjustments. Treatment of these patients is far more successful when a forum is provided for expression of their outrage, guilt, shame, distrust, and lowered self-esteem.

Just as with families of male patients, spouses and children have developed a whole range of reactions to the alcoholic behavior. These reactions can produce diminished sexual desire as a consequence of the spouse's long-term resentment and feelings of abandonment. Sexual adjustment among single women is beset by a variety of factors, which have been discussed in this book as have the special problems of lesbian alcoholics. The treatment approach with male and female homosexual alcoholics should address the alcoholism. Lovers can be included in educational programs for families and in conjoint sessions with the patient. Unless the alcoholic's sexual preference is a source of conflict, accepting it in a matter-of-fact way reduces the patient's anxiety about entering heterosexual territory—the rehabilitation center.

Drug popularity waxes and wanes. When I first became interested in treating substance abusers, my patient population was almost exclusively alcoholic, with roughly 10 percent who were physiologically addicted to sedative-hypnotics as well as alcohol, and 5 percent who abused prescription narcotics. In the 1980s there was increasing abuse of and addiction to street sedative-hypnotics, particularly Valium, and to heroin in this largely middle-class group. Now half the inpatient substance-abuse population at the hospital in which I work consists of cocaine abusers, with a consistently smaller percentage of heroin and sedative-hypnotic addicts. Alcohol remains the drug of choice for half of this population, half of whom abuse cocaine and/or are addicted to opioids as well. Many in this same group began their substance-abuse careers with daily marijuana and have continued this habit. Habitual and excessive use of these substances decreases libido and produces impotence. Hormonal mechanisms for this have been discussed in Chapter 5. These dysfunctions contradict street mythology, which often depicts the drugs as aphrodisiacs.

Bridging the research gaps between the fields of substance abuse and sexuality will greatly enhance our future knowledge in both areas.

Hormonal dysregulation produced by alcohol in male populations has been studied extensively but there is still very limited understanding of the way in which alcohol affects hormonal functioning in women. In both male and female populations, knowledge about the sexual impact of drugs other than alcohol is emerging as the popularity of these drugs increases.

Most of our previous information has been derived from retrospective studies of male populations. Large scale, prospective investigations utilizing populations of male and female substance abusers compared with controls are greatly needed.

For example, studies of identified female substance abusers in early, middle and late stages of recovery, as compared to a control population, might define the impact of substances on hormonal regulation in women. Prospective studies with control populations would, in addition, make it possible to determine whether there are differences in sexual attitudes between female substance abusers and non-abusers. Antecedent factors, such as pre-existing depression or a history of sexual victimization would have to be considered. In addition, it would be important to distinguish the sexual attitudes of women in very early stages of recovery from those of women who had been sober for at least five years in order to be certain of any true differences between substance abusing versus normal female populations.

Further elucidation of sexual attitudinal changes among men during various stages of recovery with the aid of prospective larger scale studies would be helpful.

The future, combining research efforts in the fields of substance abuse and sexuality offers rich opportunities for exploration and promises better informed patient care.

REFERENCES

Apter-Marsh, M. 1984. "The Sexual Behavior of Alcoholic Women While Drinking and During Sobriety." In *Alcoholism and Sexual Dysfunction—Issues in Clinical Management*, edited by D. J. Powell (New York: The Haworth Press).

Briddell, D. W., and G. T. Wilson. 1976. "The Effects of Alcohol and Expectancy Set on Male Sexual Arousal." *J. Abnorm. Psychol.* 85:225-34.

Cadoret, R. J., E. Troughton, and T. W. O'Gorman. 1987. "Genetics and Environmental Factors in Alcohol Abuse and Antisocial Person ality." J. Stud. Alcohol 48, no. 1:1-8.

Cloninger, C. R., M. Bohman, and S. Sigvardsson. 1981. "Inheritance of Alcohol Abuse: A Cross-Fostering Analysis of Adopted Men." *Arch. Gen. Psychiatr.* 38, no. 8:861-68.

Goodwin, D. 1985. "Alcoholism and Genetics . . . the Sins of the Fathers." *Arch. Gen. Psychiatr.* 42:171-74.

Lansky, D., and G. T. Wilson. 1981. "Alcohol, Expectations, and Sexual Arousal in Males: An Information Processing Analysis." J. Abnorm. Psychol. 90, no. 1:35-45.

Malatesta, V. J., R. H. Pollack, W. A. Wilbanks, and H. E. Adams. 1979. "Alcohol Effects on the Orgasmic-Ejaculatory Response in Human Males." *J. Sex Res.* 15, no. 2:101-7.

Masters, W., and V. Johnson. 1970. *Human Sexual Inadequacy* (Boston, MA: Little, Brown), pp. 163-68.

Wilson, G. T. 1977. "Alcohol and Human Sexual Behavior." *Behav. Res. Ther.* 15:239-52.

______. 1981. "The Effects of Alcohol on Human Sexual Behavior." In *Advances in Substance Abuse*, vol. 2 (Greenwich, CT: JAI Press), pp. 1-40.

Wilson, G. T., and D. M. Lawson. 1976. "Expectancies, Alcohol, and Sexual Arousal in Male Social Drinkers." *J. Abnorm. Psychol.* 85, no. 6:587-94.

Wilson, G. T., D. M. Lawson, and D. B. Abrams. 1978. "Effects of Alcohol on Sexual Arousal in Male Alcoholics." *J. Abnorm. Psychol.* 87, no. 6:609-16.

Wilson, G. T., and R. Niaura. 1984. "Alcohol and the Disinhibition of Sexual Responsiveness." *J. Stud. Alcohol* 45, no. 3:219-24.

Ylikahri, R., M. Huttunen, M. Harkonen, and H. Adlercreutz. 1974. "Hangover and Testosterone." *Br. Med. J.* 2:445.

Index

About the Author

CARLOTTA SCHUSTER, M.D. is Chief of the Substance Abuse Service at Silver Hill Foundation, a psychiatric hospital in New Canaan, Connecticut. She is a preceptor of psychiatric residents at St. Luke's-Roosevelt Center in New York City and is a member of the faculty of Columbia University, College of Physicians and Surgeons. Dr. Schuster is a graduate of Barnard College, and New York University, School of Medicine.

www.ingramcontent.com/pod-product-compliance
Lightning Source LLC
LaVergne TN
LVHW011512200926
848484LV00001B/26
9780275925598